The 15 Minute

Bodyweight Burn

By:

Patrick Gordon

*Disclaimer: these exercises and photos are merely suggestions of exercises that the author has found useful. You can injure yourself exercising if you don't use proper form, so please consult a professional or watch an instructional video online if you struggle with the form of an exercise. If you suffer from any conditions or health problems please consult your doctor before beginning any exercise regime.

Table of Contents:

Introduction:

One of the most amazing things I've learned about fitness over the years is how well-equipped the body is to help you get in shape. It's seriously incredible how all you need is your body and some will-power to get absolutely ripped.

As you probably know, the fitness industry is a big business and there's a lot of money and politics involved in it. Because of that, people feel so overwhelmed and don't know how to introduce a fitness plan into their lives. These big fitness businesses have popularized some myths that cause a lot of people to give up on their fitness goals before they've even tried.

Some of the myths are:
- you need to be part of a fancy gym
- hire an expensive personal trainer
- take dangerous supplements
- spend hours and hours training every week

Many people believe some or all of these myths and thus feel they'll never be able to get the body they've always wanted.

This simply isn't true.

I am here to tell you that you can make a huge difference by simply using your body and devoting 15 minutes a day. Your body is the best exercise tool you have and you can use your bodyweight to really give yourself a balanced effective workout that will be just as good if not better than a gym workout.

This book is the perfect tool to help you start an at-home bodyweight exercise program.

This book contains 100+ exercises that are:

- designed to be performed at home—no gym needed
- simple enough that anyone can do them, but targeted and efficient enough that you'll be able to target muscles and get ripped

Each exercise contains:

- pictures of the exercise
- Detailed instructions on how to perform the exercise
- Most exercises have a **Best practices** section—extra tips to help you really nail the movement
- Some exercises contain a: **For added emphasis** section. This is for those of you that want a bigger challenge. You've already mastered the basic exercise? This shows you how to make it harder and more challenging meaning that you'll achieve even bigger gains.
- **Breathing instructions:** one of the most helpful aspects of exercise is knowing when to inhale and exhale. If you follow my instructions, you'll be amazed at how much easier the exercise is and how you'll be able to power through those difficult last reps
- **Primary and Secondary Muscle groups:** this really helps you understand what muscle group you're targeting by this exercise. Through this you'll be able to plan a balanced workout routine.

This book contains great exercises for:

- Legs, hamstrings, quadriceps, calves
- Biceps, triceps, full arms, forearms
- Abs, core, obliques
- Shoulders
- Chest
- Back, delts, lats, lower back

Helpful equipment: this is a list of some equipment it may be helpful to have in your home to make these exercises even more effective. However, none of this is strictly necessary, and 95% of these exercises can be performed with no equipment or with ordinary stuff you have in your house.

- Chin up bar
- Exercise bands
- Dumbells
- Ab Wheel Roller
- Large inflatable yoga ball

As you can see, this is COMPREHENSIVE. It gets every muscle you need to focus on. Now there are no more excuses. All you need is your body, this book and 15 minutes a day. Anyone can do that, and once you start seeing results, you are going to be asking yourself why you haven't been following this approach to exercise your whole life.

I hope you get great use out of this book and I really hope it helps you crush your fitness goals and get closer to the body you've always wanted.

Section 1: Leg Exercises

1). Standing Calf Raise:

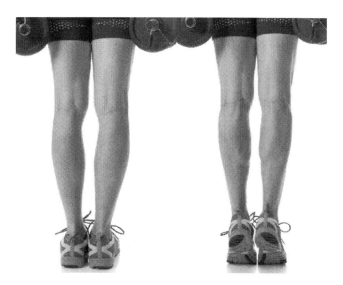

How:

1. Stand upright with arms at your sides, feet flat.

2. Lift your heals off the ground slowly squeezing your calf muscles. Raise your heels as high as you can and then hold for a few seconds

3. Slowly lower your heels back to the floor.

Breathing:

1. Exhale as you raise your heals and hold.
2. Inhale as you return your heels to the ground.

Best Practice:

1. A simple way to really feel a burn with this exercise is by standing with your feet halfway on a step (any step or stairs in your house) with heels hanging off. You get better Range of motion which makes for a better muscle building exercise.

For Added Emphasis:

Use dumbells and hold them at your sides while you do the calf raises. You will build muscle much more quickly this way.

Try: 4 sets of 20 reps, as the exercise gets easier, try it with dumbbells to increase the resistance and make it harder.

Primary Muscle Group: Calf Muscles

2). Wall Sit:

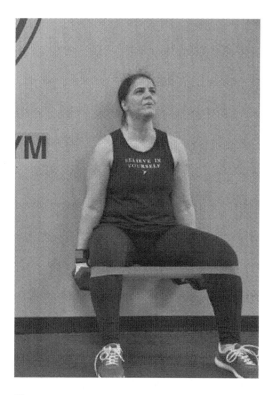

How :

1. Find an open spot of sturdy wall.
2. Stand with your back to the wall legs about shoulder width apart.
3. Slide your back down the wall and move your feet out until you are in a sitting position bending your knees until your legs make a 90 degree angle and your thighs are parallel with the ground
4. Keep your back straight against the wall hold the position for the full set, and then return to a standing position

Breathing:

Concentrate on keeping your breathing deep and steady, especially as your quads start to burn.

Best Practice:

- It helps to have something for your mind to focus on. Try reading a book or listening to a podcast while doing this so your mind can focus on something other than the burning in your legs.
- Keep back straight against the wall, if you lean forward you could hurt your back and or knees.

Try: *4 sets at 60 seconds per set.*

As you practice and the exercise becomes easier, you can add weight to your lap (a heavy dictionary or something) and try to always be increasing the amount of time you can hold the position.

Primary Muscle Group: Quadriceps

Secondary: Hamstrings, Lower Back, Full Body

3). Air Squats:

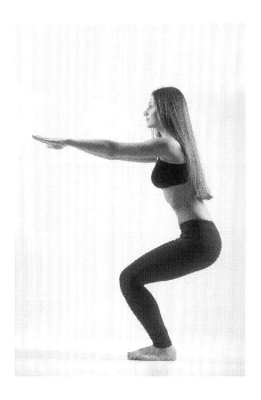

How:

1. Stand straight up on the floor with your feet slightly less than shoulder width apart. Make sure your toes are pointed slightly outward instead of straight ahead. Let your arms hang at your sides, and push your chest out with your back slightly arched inward.

2. Bend at your knees pushing your butt out. Try to keep your shins straight and only move your body from the knees up. Center your wait on your heels firmly and don't rock on your feel or roll forward onto the balls of your feet.

3. Keep bending pushing your butt backward and lowering it as far as you can. Keep going past the point where your thighs are parallel to the ground.

4. Keep your knees slightly pointing out, do not let them draw in (you can hurt your knees this way).

5. Slowly start to rise back up. Pulling your butt back in and pushing off your heels straighten up until you are at the starting position.

6. Push yourself just a bit beyond a normal straight standing position so you're pushing your chest out, arching your back inward and squeezing your butt firmly planted on your heels.

7. That's the completed exercise and you'll want to repeat this for the number of reps in your set.

Breathing:

1. Exhale as you bend and start to squat
2. Hold your breath for the first burst as you just start to push your body back up
3. Exhale as you straighten back up and return to the start position

Best Practice:

1. Squats are one of the most useful and effective exercises you can do, but they are also tricky and one of most difficult exercises to perform accurately. Watch a lot of videos online so you can see other people doing the form and have someone who knows what they're doing, watch you and critique your form.

2. Squat sideways in front of a mirror so you can see your side profile. This will help you monitor and improve your form
3. Push your arms out straight in front of you as you squat. This will help you keep your balance and keep your weight centered on your heels.

For Added Emphasis:

1. Squat holding a dumbbell or a kettlebell. Do not try this until you've mastered the form.

Try:

Dropsets, 4 sets as follows: Set 1: 40 squats, Set 2: 30 Squats, Set 3: 20 Squats, Set 4: 10 squats.

Increase reps as you improve.

Primary Muscle Group: Hamstrings and Quadriceps

Secondary: Lower Back, Glutes, Full Body

4). Pistol Squats:

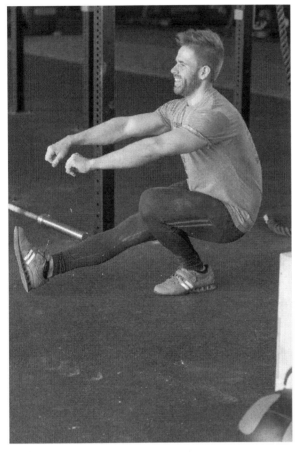

How:

1.   Follow All the same instructions for regular squats (see previous exercise for detailed instructions), but instead you'll be squatting on one leg.
2.   As you start to squat, push one of your legs and both of your arms straight out in front of you for balance.
3.   As you start to raise your body back up and straighten your leg, pull your outstretched leg in slowly until you are standing on both feet at the start position.
4.   Then, repeat and switch legs.

Breathing:

1.   Inhale as you lower yourself into the squat
2.   Exhale as you straighten back up

Best Practices:

1. You will need something to hold onto for balance when you first try this exercise. Try squatting next to a chair and holding onto it with your outstretched hand for balance.
2. When your're able to do the exercise well while holding onto something, you can progress to squatting onto a stool or step. This will give you a reference point and a pushoff point. Instead of hanging onto something for support, do a one legged squat until your butt touches the stool or step and push yourself back off
3. Until you've mastered these two variations, don't try to just do the unsupported pistol squat.

For Added Emphasis: This is one of the most difficult exercises you can master, so start with the two variations listed under Best Practices. Once you've mastered those, move onto the full unsupported pistol squat. Once you can do that without help, you should feel very accomplished because many people cannot perform this exercise.

Try: *4 Sets of 10 squats. Once you've improves, move onto drop sets of 40, 30, 20, 10 etc.*

Primary Muscle Group: Hamstrings and Quadriceps

Secondary: Lower Back, Glutes, Full Body

5). Scissor Jumps (Squat Jumps):

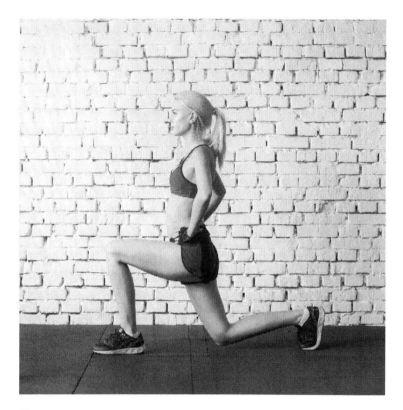

How:

1. Start in a standing position, feet together, arms hanging at your sides.

2. Lower your right leg bending at the knee until you are in a lunge position (as pictured). Your left leg will bend at the knee. Your left thigh should be parallel to the floor and your right thigh perpendicular (see picture)

3. Immediately spring upward bringing your legs together and land in an opposing lunge position. (With your right leg close

to the ground (left quad parallel to the ground). This basically means you land in the starting position but with your legs in opposite positions from how you started).

4. Repeat this movement (spring back up) and land back in the original lunge position. Keep repeating for the duration of the set.

Breathing: Inhale as you lower your body into the lunge, then hold your breath a moment as you push your body back up from the lunge position and exhale as you spring upwards.

Best Practices:

- For newcomers the coordination of this exercise can be tricky, and it may be difficult to complete a set. If you find it overly difficult, try doing alternating speed lunges where you lunge with one leg, then reverse back into a standing position and lunge on the other leg. Repeat as quickly as possible without pausing
- As this gets easier, start springing from lunge to lunge

For Added Emphasis:

Lunge with 5 lb dumbells in each hand. Increase the weight for even more of a strain.

Try: *60 Seconds of continuous lunges, 60 seconds rest. Do 3 sets of this.*

Primary Muscle Groups: Quads, Calves

Secondary Muscle Group: Glutes, Hamstrings (Full Lower Body)

---

6). Step Up Knee-Ups:

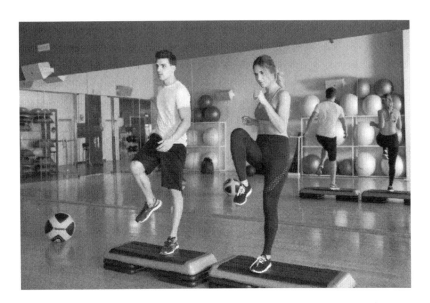

How:

1. Stand in front of a step or a low bench or a sturdy flat stool.
2. Step with one foot onto the stool and bring your other leg up raising your knee up until it's parallel with the floor (or higher). Raise your knee as high as you can get it.
3. Lower your knee and step down from the stool with both feet, then switch legs. Step onto the step with the other leg and raise the knee on your first leg.

Breathing:

Exhale as you raise your knee, Inhale as you lower your knee and step down.

Best Practices:

- Get your knee as high as you can. Getting it to the point where your thigh is parallel with the floor is a minimum.
- Move fast and try to increase your speed each time

For Added Emphasis: hold 5 lb. dumbells in each hand with your arms straight at your sides as you perform this exercise.

Try: *60 seconds of as many as you can do, 60 Seconds rest. Do 3 sets. As you improve, increase your speed and decrease your rest time to 30 seconds.*

Primary Muscle Group: Quads

Secondary Muscles: Hamstrings, Calves, Glutes

7). Side Lunge:

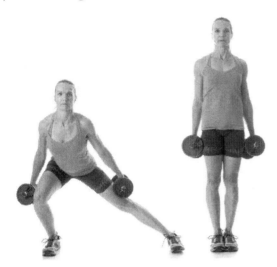

How:

1. Stand up straight with your feet together.
2. Step to the left moving your left foot several feet to the left bending at the knee while keeping your right foot planted.
3. Lower yourself into the side lunge straightening your right leg and bending your left. Squat down as low as you can squeezing your glutes.
4. Raise yourself back up into a standing position moving your left foot back to the starting position. Then repeat to the right, lunging onto the right foot.

Breathing: Inhale as you lower yourself into the lunge, exhale as you push yourself back into a standing position.

Best Practices:

- Move slowly. Do not try to speed through this exercise. Be smooth and fluid with your movements.
- Try to squeeze your glutes as you lunge and try to go as low as you can

For Added Emphasis:

- Hold 10-20 lb. dumbells in each hand as you lunge. Keep your arms straight at your sides.

Try:60 seconds lunging alternating to the left and right. 30 seconds rest. Do 4 sets.

Primary Muscle: Glutes

Secondary Muscles: Quads, hamstrings.

8). Glute Lift

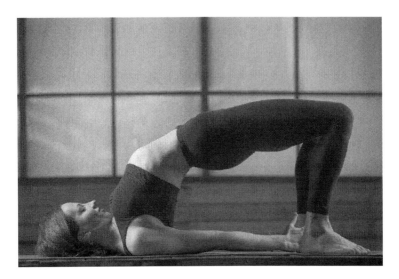

How:

1. Lie flat on the floor on your back and keep your hands at your sides & knees bent.
2. Slowly lift your butt off the floor keeping your shoulders on the ground.
3. Keep in this position for a second, but remember when you lift your butt your body will remain in a straight line.
4. Flex your glutes and really straing and push with your butt
5. Come back to the starting position and repeat.

Breathing:

- Exhale as you lift your butt off the ground.
- Inhale as you go back to the starting position.

Best practices:

- This exercise will tone your glutes and stabilize your spine.

- Glute lift is one of the most effective butt building or body shaping workouts.
- When you perform this workout you must keep your core & glutes tight.
- And maintain the whole body in a controlled manner and bend knees at 45 degrees.

Try:

- Do at least 2 to 3 sets of 10 reps and increase the reps when you get enough strength.

Primary Muscles: Glutes

Secondary Muscles: Hamstrings, Core

9). Mountain Climbers:

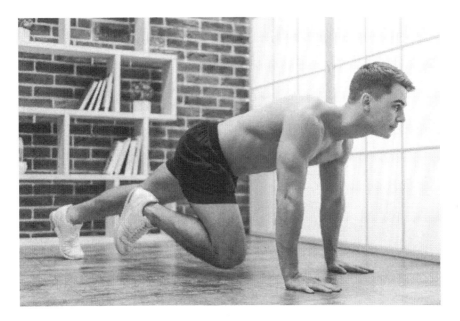

How:

1. Get into pushup position (body parallel to the ground arms straight, back straight.
2. While keeping your left leg planted and straight, move your right foot straight inward bending at the knee until your thigh is almost perpendicular to the ground and your leg makes a 90 degree angle.
3. Touch your toe to the ground at this point and return your leg to starting position. Then repeat with the left leg while keeping your right leg planted.

Breathing:

This is a continuous exercise so you may find it difficult to coordinate your breathing. Some may find it easier to exhale as they move their leg inward and inhale as they move it back to start position. I prefer to focus on just taking very deep controlled slow breaths throughout.

Best Practices:

- Keep your back straight or slightly arched outward.
- Try to get your knee as far up as possible touching your toe as far up the floor as you can
- Be fast and continuous. This exercise is meant to be vigorous and continuous.

Try:

60 seconds continuous as fast as you can, and 30 seconds rest. Do 4 sets.

Primary Muscle: Core

Secondary: Quads

10). Static Lunge:

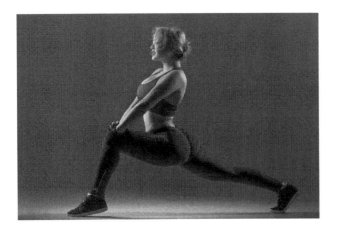

How:

1. Start by standing up straight with your feet hips-breadth apart.
2. Tighten your abs and keep your back straight by looking straight ahead.
3. Lunge your right foot forward and left foot in a back position.
4. Bend your both knees until your back knee comes just near to the floor.
5. Hold this position several seconds
6. Slowly go back to the starting point by pressing your right heel.
7. And repeat this exercise

Breathing:

- Inhale when you lunge
- Exhale when you return to the starting position

Best Practices:

- The lunge simultaneously works for the numerous muscle groups and helps you to lose weight.
- Try to keep your balance on both feet.

Try:

- Do 2 to 4 sets of 6 to 10 repetitions per leg that is enough during a strength training routine. Hold for 5-10 seconds per lunge

Primary Muscles: Quads, Hamstrings, Glutes

Secondary Muscles: Abs

11). Sumo Squat:

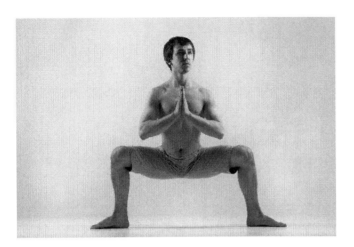

How:

1. Start standing in a wide posture as your toes pointed outwards.
2. Bend your knees while lowering yourself and pushing your hips back. Almost like you're sitting into something.
3. When your thighs are parallel to the floor, return and repeat the exercise.
4. As you're returning to start position, you almost want to swing your hips up and push your groin forward to make sure you're getting the full motion

Breathing:

- Inhale when you squat.
- Exhale when you return to the starting point.

Best practices:

- Keep in mind that when you perform Sumo Squat you should keep your back straight, knees in line with your toes and Abs tight.

- Sumo Squat strengthens your lower body and you can also perform this by combining flutter kick squats & jump squats, it burns more calories.
- Sumo Squat will be challenging for beginners because you are putting your body in a new position and you need stability. So just move slowly until you get it

Try:

- Add 2 to 3 sets of 15 to 20 reps of Sumo Squats. Do regularly and increase the challenge as you get perfection.

Primary Muscles: Inner thighs, Glutes

Secondary Muscles: Calves, Hip flexor, Quads, Hamstrings

12). Back Kick Exercise:

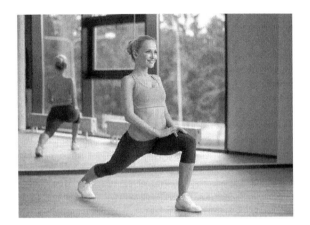

How:

1. Begin with your feet hip-breadth apart.
2. Take a step forward on your right leg and lunge.
3. Come back to the initial position and kick back your right leg, squeezing the glutes.
4. Go back to the starting posture and do the same technique with the left leg.
5. So you're basically lunging forward, then backward

Breathing:

- Inhale when you lunge.
- Exhale when you kick back.

Best Practices:

- Throughout this exercise, keep your back straight and face front.
- Keep your core engaged

Try:

- Do 2 to 3 sets of 30 seconds to 1 minute continuous and increase the challenge after a time.

Primary Muscles: Quads, Hip flexors, Glutes

Secondary Muscles: Abs, Calves, Hamstrings

13). Jump Squats:

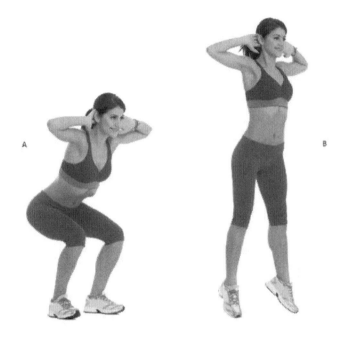

How :

1. Start by standing with feet shoulder-width apart, toes pointing out.
2. Squeeze your hips back and slightly bend your knees. (In a squat posture).
3. Jump straight up by pushing off from your heels.
4. Land with your knees, slightly bent and return into the squat pose.
5. Repeat until the desired sets completed.

Breathing:

- Throughout this workout keep your breathing pattern natural and steady.
- Exhale when you jump.

Best Practices:

- keep your back in a perfect position by keeping your hips back & chest up.
- Always put pressure on your heels, but never extend your knees beyond your toes.
- Landing softly on your toes or feet's balls and slightly bend your knees.

Try:

- 2 sets of 8 to 15 repetitions, but make sure keep in a perfect form.

Primary Muscles: Hip flexors, Glutes, Quads

Secondary Muscles: Lower back, Abs, Calves, Hamstrings

14). Leg Raise Bridge:

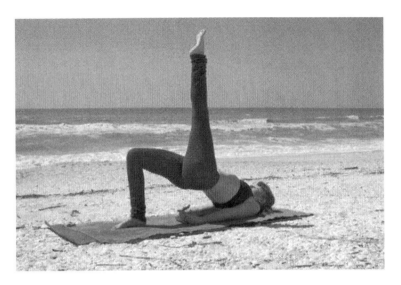

How:

1. Lie straight on an exercise mat and keep your arms by your sides, knees bent.
2. Keep your feet flat on the floor.
3. Lift your right leg off the ground and raise hips simultaneously by pushing off your left heel.
4. Keep your hips are in a straight line with your chest (diagonal).
5. Hold this posture for a few seconds and lower your hips.
6. Repeat the same process on another leg.

Breathing:

- Exhale when you raise the hips.

Best Practices:

- Make sure your glutes and Abs remains tight throughout the process.

- Keep your upper body in a comfortable and neutral posture.

Try:

- Perform 3 sets of 8 to 12 reps for each leg

Primary Muscles: Glutes

Secondary Muscles: Knee extensors, Core, Hip flexors

15). Single Leg Calf Raise:

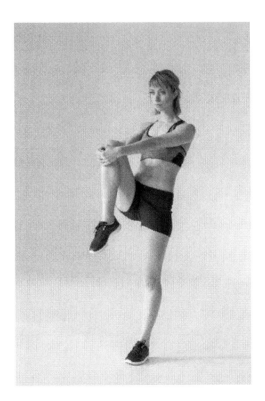

How:

1. Follow the same instructions as the standing calf raise (see exercise 1) but implement the variations in the following steps.

There are two ways to do this exercise:

2. **The easier way:** lift your left foot off the ground and raise it behind you bending at the knee until your leg is at a 90 degree angle (shin parallel to the ground behind you).

OR

The harder way: raise your knee in front of you until your thigh is parallel to the ground (leg at a 90 degree angle raised in front of you, see picture)

3. Rise up onto the ball of your right foot, which is planeted on the ground and squeeze your calf muscle.
4. Lower yourself as far as you can arching your foot downward before repeating.

Breathing:

Exhale as you rise onto the balls of your feet and squeeze your calf muscle. Inhale as you lower yourself back down.

Best Practices:

- If you do the harder version, you will get a quad workout for your elevated leg while you are working your calf on your other leg.

Try:*25 reps on each leg, 3 sets each.*

Primary Muscle: Calf

Secondary Muscle(s): Quads (if you do the harder version)

___

16). Side Plank Leg Raise:

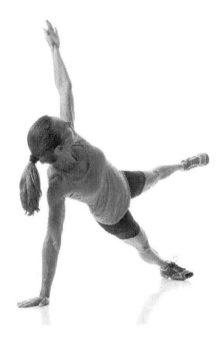

How:

1. Lay on your right side
2. Keep your elbow straight under your shoulders and put your forearm on the ground.
3. Lift your hips off the floor keeping your whole body in a straight diagonal line from head to toes.
4. Engage your core and raise your body into the side plank position keeping your body equally balanced between the feet and elbow. (This is starting point).
5. Raise your top leg to hip height, but keep your leg straight and hold your leg in this posture for a few seconds.
6. Now slowly lower your leg. Perform the indicated number or reps, then switch sides.

Breathing:

- Breathe in when you raise the leg.
- Breathe out when you lower the leg.

Best practices:

- complete all moves in a controlled and slow movement.

Try:

- 8 to 12 repetitions in your workout routine, 3 sets each leg

Primary Muscles: Obliques, full leg

Secondary Muscles: Glutes, Hip abductors, Shoulder, Abdominal

17). Butt Kicks:

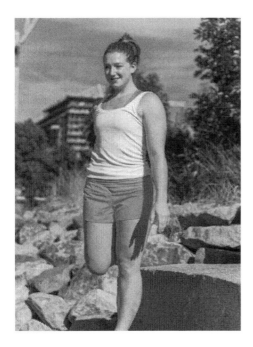

How:

1. Begin standing straight on your feet and keep your feet shoulder-width apart.
2. Keep your head facing forward and bring one heel off the ground.
3. Start kicking backwards toward towards your butt
4. Repeat and switch to the other side.

Breathing:

- Throughout the exercise, maintain stable & steady speed.
- Exhale as you kick back.

Best Practices:

- If you are a beginner and can't get total contact with your backside, then patiently develop your performance over time.
- Your arms will remain close to your torso and bent elbows at 90 degrees angle.

Try:

- complete 2 to 3 sets of 30 seconds to 1 minute continuous alternating legs every time.

Primary Muscles: Glutes, Hamstrings

Secondary Muscles: Arms, Legs, Abs, Back

18). Knee Ups

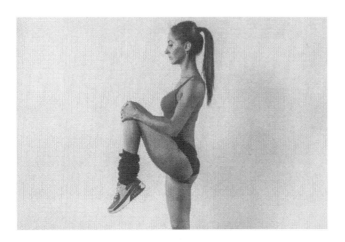

How:

1. Stand with your feet together, back straight.
2. Slowly drive your right knee up until it forms a 90 degree angle and your thigh is parallel with the floor.
3. Lower your leg rapidly and switch legs and do the same with the other.
4. Repeat for indicated set

Breathing:

- Exhale as you're raising your knee, inhale as you're lowering it.

Best Practices:

- When performing this exercise, keep your shoulders back, chest open and face front.

Try:

- 3 sets, 30 seconds continuous alternating legs each time.

Primary Muscles: Quads

Secondary Muscles: Glutes, Hamstrings

SECTION 2: Ab Exercises

1). Leg Raise:

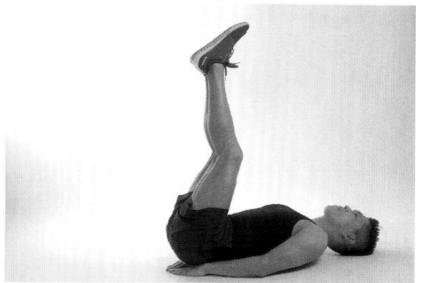

How:

1. Lay flat on the ground (preferably on a mat or on a carpeted floor).
2. Elevate your feet a few inches off the ground, keeping your feet together.
3. Raise them up keeping your legs straight as far as you can (try to get your legs to form a 90 degree angle with your body) until your legs are vertical.
4. Hold that position while clenching your abdominal muscles, and hold for 3-5 seconds

5. Lower your legs keeping the together until you're back to a few inches off the ground, but do not rest your legs on the ground until you've completed the set.
6. Repeat until the set is completed.

Breathing:

Exhale as you raise your legs, and hold your breath briefly while pausing when your legs are fully raised. Inhale as you lower your legs.

Best Practices:

- Arch your back slightly and curl your upper body up a little to really push the strain on your abs.
- Keep your legs as straight as possible and try to lift with your abs instead of your legs

Try:*Set 1: 60 seconds continuous, 60 seconds rest, Set 2: 45 seconds continuous, 30 seconds rest, Set 3: 30 seconds continuous, 30 seconds rest.*

Primary Muscle Group: Abs

Secondary Muscles: Legs

2). Bicycle Abs:

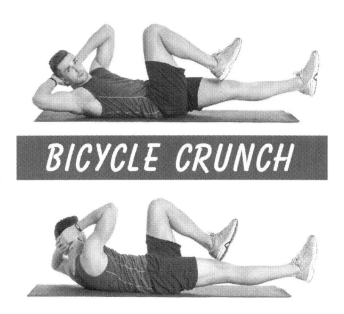

How:

1. Lie flat on the floor (on a mat or carpet).
2. Raise yourself up onto your lower back arching your back outward and curling your head and shoulders up so they're not touching the ground.
3. Raise your legs off the ground as well so the only part of your body that's touching the ground is your lower back and butt. Put your hands behind your head bending your elbows.
4. Move your legs in a circular motion bending at the knee as if riding a bicycle keeping your toes pointed.
5. Simultaneously move your upper body forward towards your knees touching your left bent elbow to your right bent knee, and then your right bent elbow to your to your left bent knee. (hands still behind head).

6. Clench your abs and slightly rotate your body from side to side as you stretch to touch elbow to knee.

Breathing:

Since this is a continuous burn, just focus on taking controlled deep breaths. Do not pant or let yourself get short on breath.

BestPractices:

- The coordination of this exercise can be difficult, but it's really important to do it correctly otherwise you may not be actually effectively working your abs. Watch videos of people performing the exercise and practice keeping your balance and keeping your shoulders and legs off the ground

Try: *30 Seconds continuous, 20 seconds rest. Do 3 sets*

Primary Muscle: Abs

Secondary Muscle: Obliques, Core, Legs

3). Leg Raise Figure 8:

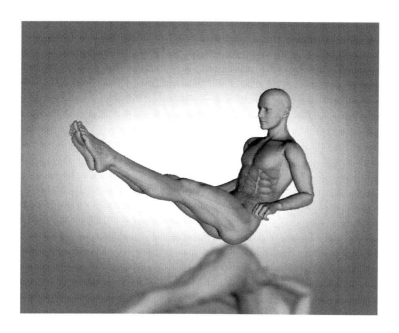

How:

1. Sit on the floor with your legs extended in front of you, feet together,
2. Lift your legs off the ground keeping your feet together and rock back onto your lower back keeping your shoulders off the ground.
3. Keep your toes pointed and moved your feet in a figure 8 in the air (your feet should be about 12-18 inches off the ground)

Breathing: keep deep, steady breaths throughout the exercise—do not pant or take shallow breaths

Best Practices: Tighten your abs and try to focus your attention and strain on your abs as opposed to your quads or legs.

Try: 30 seconds clockwise, 30 seconds rest, then 30 seconds counterclockwise. If you want to make it more challenging, omit the rest period.

Primary Muscle Group: Abdominals

Secondary: Obliques, quadriceps

4). V-ups:

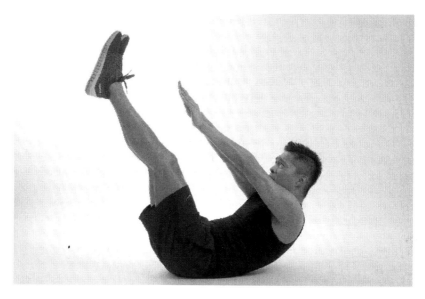

How:

1. Lie flat on your back on a mat or on carpeted floor.
2. Simultaneously raise your upper body and legs stretching your arms in front of you for balance.
3. Keep your legs and back straight as your body forms a "V" or "U" shape, while you stay balanced on your lower back.
4. Clench your abs as you curl your body into a "V," then lower your legs and upper body until you're flat on your back again.
5. Repeat for the rest of the set.

Breathing:

Exhale as you curl your body up, and inhale as you lower your body back to start position. (You may want to hold your breath at the height of the exercise while you're clenching your abs).

Best Practice:

- Stretch your arms out straight in front of you to help with balance (reach for your feet)

Try: *25 reps, 3 sets (as the exercise becomes easier, increase reps and/or sets*

Primary Muscle: Abs
Secondary Muscles: Legs, Core

5). Leg Lifts:

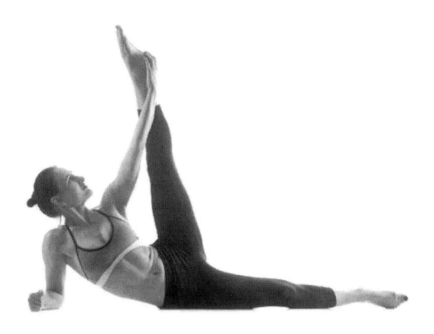

How:

1. Lie on the floor on your side and keep legs stacked on top of each other, feet together & legs completely extended.
2. Raise your left leg and keeping it as straight as possible
3. Pause for 2 seconds and lower the leg.
4. Switch the side and repeat.

Breathing:

- Breathe out as you lift your leg.

- Breathe in as you lower your leg.

Best Practices:

- Keep your core tight and body in a stable posture.

Try:

- Perform 8 to 10 res per set, 3 sets per side.

Primary Muscles: Abdominals, Obliques

Secondary Muscles: Thighs, Hips, Glutes, Core

---

6). Leg Raise Circles, clockwise and counter clockwise:

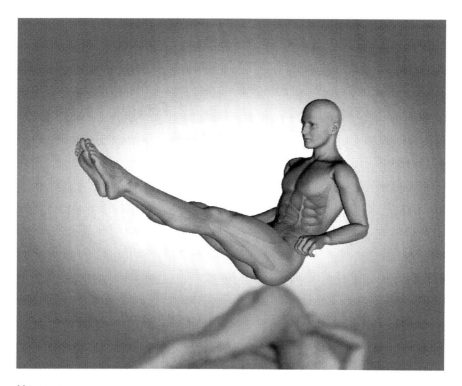

How to:

1. Lie flat on your back on a mat or carpeted floor.
2. Raise your legs about 6 inches off the ground keeping your feet together and legs straight and prop yourself up slightly on your elbows.
3. Move your feet together in a clockwise circle in the air (about 1.5 feet wide). Keep your toes pointed
4. Continue moving your feet in circles clenching your abs throughout.
5. After that set, pause and switch direction and start moving your feet in the opposite (counterclockwise direction).

Breathing:

Since this is a continuous burn, just focus on taking steady deep measured breaths.

For Added Emphasis:

Instead of propping yourself on your elbows, simply raise your upper body a few inches off the ground and hold and let your abs to the extra work.

Try:30 seconds clockwise, then immediately switch to 30 seconds counterclockwise without resting your legs. Do 2 sets in each direction.

Primary Muscle: Abs

Secondary Muscle: Legs, Core, Obliques

---

7). Vertical Inverted Leg raise

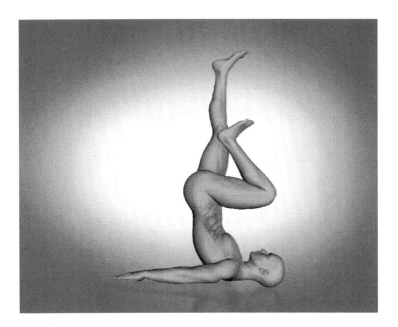

How:

1. Lie straight on your back keeping hands at your sides or under your glutes if you need the extra support.
2. Lift both legs directly flexing your hips & knees and keep your right leg straight & left leg just bent above the knee. Hold briefly

3. Then raise your bent leg straightening it out until its perfectly perpendicular with the ground, while simutaneaously bending your left leg at the knee.
4. Repeat until completed desired set.

Breathing:
Inhale while moving legs, exhale while holding

Best Practices:
- Keep your shoulders planted on the floor and neck down.
- Your Abs should remain engaged in all the time as it's focused on your abs.

Try:
If you are beginner then start with 2 to 3 sets of 8 to 12 repetitions. As you improve, increase the number until you're capable to complete 3 sets of 25 to 50 repetitions.

Primary Muscles: Abs
Secondary Muscles: Lower back

8). Ab Wheel Roll:

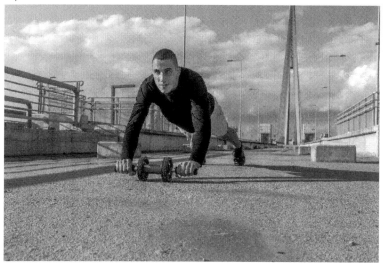

How:

1. Kneel down on the floor and grasp the ab wheel roll firmly overhanded and place it on the ground in front of you
2. Abs tight, not sagging and slowly roll the wheel or ab roller squeezing your glutes and abs.
3. Roll it out extending your body and try to keep your knees off the ground.
4. Keep roller in front of your body and hips extended.
5. Must focus on your core and stretching your arms until your nose hardly almost touches the floor.

6. Take a reverse movement to come back to the starting point.

Breathing:

- Inhale as you rolled the wheel.
- Exhale as you roll back to the starting position.

Best Practices:

- Perform it slowly and keep your Abs tight throughout the exercise.
- If it's too difficult, do it kneeling until you've mastered the form

Try:

- Do 3 sets of 8 to 12 repetitions.

Primary Muscles: Abs

Secondary Muscles: Lower back, Glutes, Lats

9). Ball Crunch:

NOTE: you will need a large yoga ball or something similar in order to properly do this exercise.

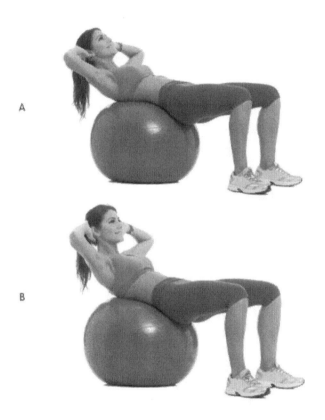

How:

1. Lie with your back on the ball feet planted in front of you, knees bent at a 90 degree angle.
2. Roll backwards on the ball so that your upper body is hanging off the ball and you are balanced mainly on your lower back.

3. Slowly curl your upper body inwards and upwards towards your knees squeezing your abs as hard as you can.
4. Lower your upper body back to start position then repeat.

Breathing:

Exhale as you curl upwards, inhale as you lower back to start position.

For Added Emphasis:

- Place your hands behind your head bending your elbows and really pull with your abs
- Try a variation where you rotate your left elbow to right knee and right elbow to left knee (similar to bicycle ab exercise).

Try: 2 *sets to failure (this means do as many as you possibly can until you physically cannot continue). Keep track of how many you do each time and make sure every time you are improving.*

Primary Muscle Group: Abs

10). Flutter Kick:

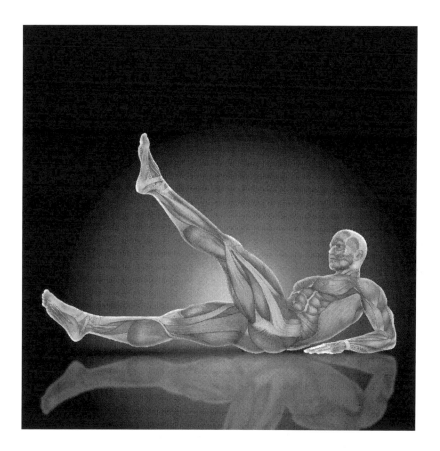

How:

1. Lie flat on the floor keeping your hands or elbows on the floor, palms down
2. Raise your back off the floor and keep head straight.
3. Lift your legs a few inches off the ground and then raise one of the legs higher so it's 12-16 inches off the ground.

4. Return slowly so the legs are together a few inches off the ground and Repeat with other leg.

Breathing:

- Throughout the exercise, breathe slowly and flex your abs.

Best practices:

- Keep Your chin off your chest, legs straight and head in a neutral posture.
- Keep your shoulders off the ground and try to balance on your glutes and lower back
-

Try:

- Do at least 2 to 3 sets of 30 seconds continuous

Primary Muscles: Abs

Secondary Muscles: Quads, Hip flexors

11). In and Outs:

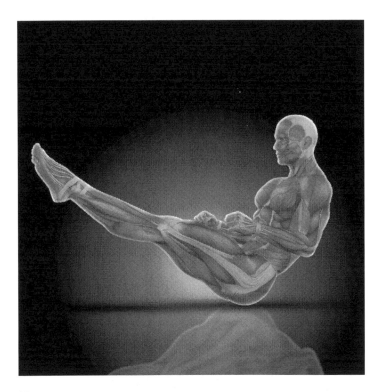

How:

1. Sit on a flat bench leaning slightly back balancing on your butt and lower back with your legs outstretched and slightly elevated.
2. Plant your hands on either side of your body next to your hips
3. for support.
4. Bring your legs in bending at the knee until you're practically hugging your legs.
5. Then kick your legs back out straightening them back to starting point
6. Repeat

Breathing:

Exhale as you draw your legs into your chest, inhale as you straighten your legs back out and return to start position.

Best Practices:

- Point your toes and arch your feet
- Pull with your abs and not your legs

For Added Emphasis:

Instead of planting your hands by your hips, cross them over your chest and make your abs do the work of holding up your upper body.

Try:*Set 1: 40, Set 2: 30, Set 3: 20, Set 4: 10*

Primary Muscle: Abs

12). Weighted Situp:

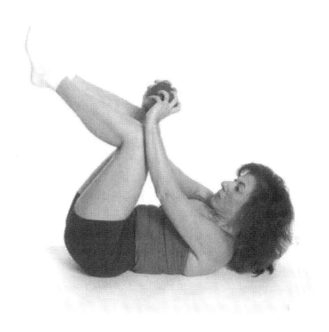

How to do:

1. Lie down on the floor keeping your knees, back, and feet straight on the mat.
2. Grab a small ball or any other objective tightly.
3. Gradually raise your chest and sit up.
4. Come back to the starting position by bending down one vertebrae at the time.
5. Repeat the process for recommended reps.

Breathing:

- Inhale when you lift your torso.
- Exhale when you slowly come back to the starting position.

Best practice:

- In this exercise, you should Keep Abs engaged and neck, chest, shoulders & back in a relaxed position.
- This exercise will help you in toning & sculpt your abdomen and reduce your waist.
- Sit up exercise targets your abs and also toned your hips, flexor & torso.

Try:

- Perform 2 to 3 sets of 12 to 16 reps and increase with rolling down your back.

Primary Muscles: Abs

Secondary Muscles: Hip flexors

13). Standing Knee to Elbow:

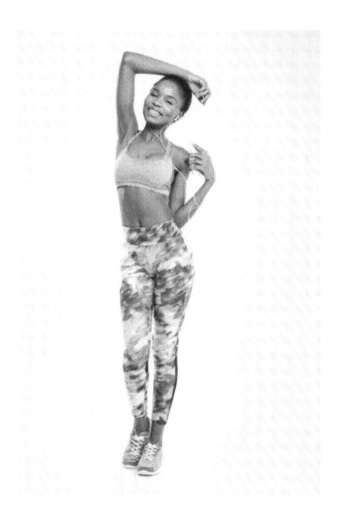

How:

1. Start by standing up straight feet hip-width apart.
2. Keep your hands behind your head, raise your knee and slightly bend your right leg.
3. Turn your chest to the right side and move your right knee to the left elbow.

4. Return & Repeat the process on the opposite side and keep on changing the sides until set completed.

Breathing:

- Keep smooth & steady breathing.
- Inhale as you bring knee to elbow.
- Exhale when you return to starting point.

Best Practices:

- As your body keeps a working movement, it helps to increase heart rate and burn more body fat.
- When doing this exercise, keep your back straight; engage your core muscles and neck in a relaxed position.

Try:

- Do 30 seconds to 1-minute sets and move as fast as you can in a perfect form, do 2-3 sets

Primary Muscles: Obliques, Hip flexors, Abs

Secondary Muscles: Thighs, Quads, Glutes

---

14). L Sit

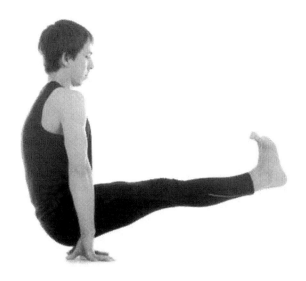

How:

1. Start to sit in a pike seated pose on the floor and keep your legs straight in front of you.
2. Put your hands on the ground near your hips, palms down and arms fully extended, locked.
3. Your arms remain locked at the elbow as you lift your butt off the ground with shoulders by forcing your hands against the ground.
4. Keep your core tight and raise your legs off to the floor, but keep your legs straight and together extended in front of you.
5. When you are up, keep your hips ahead of your hands, feet up off to the floor.
6. Hold this posture for preferred time.

Breathing:

- In this exercise, you need deep breathing.
- Inhale as you lift your butt
- Exhale as you lower your body to the floor.

Best Practice:

- If it's too difficult, try it with your heels on the ground and raise your butt off the ground instead of your whole body. You'll still want to keep your arms straight and locked, you'll just allow your heels to touch the ground of added support.

Try:

- Perform 3 sets of 10 to 12 reps in 30 seconds.

Primary Muscles: Abs

Secondary Muscles: Quads, Triceps, Forearm, Hip Flexors.

---

15). Six Inches:

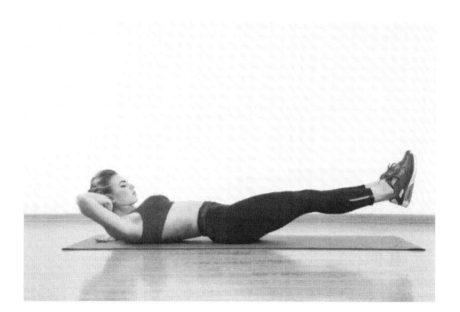

How:

1. Lie down on the floor on your back.
2. Completely extend your body and keep your legs straight.
3. Your toes pointed upward.
4. Keep your hands at your sides which give extra support to your back.
5. Keeping your abs tight and raise your feet six inches off the floor.
6. Hold in this position and count 3 to 5 counts and return to the starting point and repeat the same process.

Breathing:

- Keep stable and regular breathing throughout the workout.
- Inhale while you put down your legs
- Exhale when you lift your legs

Best practices:

- Throughout the exercise have focused, smooth and controlled movements.
- This exercise will be good for tightening and shaping your lower abs and give you a flatter stomach.
- It will also stabilize your core strength, but you need to do twice in a week.

Try:

- Do at least 10 repetitions.

Primary Muscles: Abs

Secondary Muscles: Glutes, hips

Section 3: Oblique Exercises

1). Side Crunch:

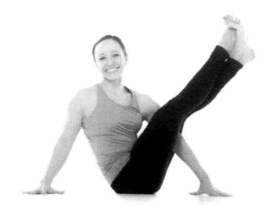

How:

1. Lie on your side with your body rotated slightly inward towards your stomach.
2. Move your upper body and legs inward keeping both straight until your body forms a 45 degree angle.
3. Prop your upper body up slightly on your elbow and place your other hand behind your head elbow bent.
4. Keep your feet together and legs as straight as possible.

5. Crunch sideways bringing your legs up and curling your upper body up trying to touch your elbow to your feet.
6. Lower your legs to star position but do not let them touch the floor until the set has been completed. Repeat.
7. After the set is completed, roll onto your other side and do the exercise from that side.

Breathing:

Exhale as you raise your legs, Inhale as you lower them

Best Practices:

- Move around until you really feel the burn in your obliques and stick to that position.
- Squeeze your obliques when your legs are fully raised.

Try: *15 reps on your left and 15 on your right. 3 sets per side.*

Primary Muscle: Obliques

Secondary Muscle: Abs

2). Side Plank:

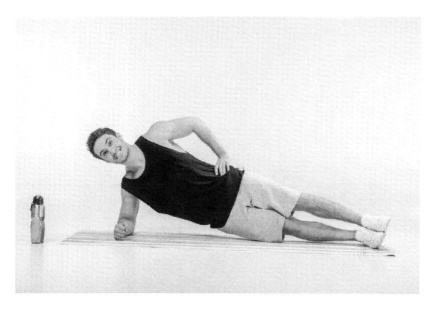

How:

1. Get into pushup position and lower yourself onto your elbows (your whole body off the ground).
2. Roll onto your left side so you are supported by your left elbow. Stretch your right arm straight up to the ceiling for balance.
3. Keep your body as straight as possible. And clench your core.
4. Hold for the duration of the set. Then go back to pushup position and rotate to your other side and repeat.

Breathing:

This is a continuous burn, so just take controlled deep breaths throughout. Keep your breaths consistent and slow.

Best Practices:

- Arch your back slightly and squeeze your obliques for a full burn
- Don't let your hips sag, try to keep your body in a perfectly straight diagonal line from your head to your toes.

Try: *60 seconds plank, 30 seconds rest, then switch sides and repeat. Do 3 sets each side.*

Primary Muscle Group: Obliques

Secondary Muscle Group: Core

3). Pushup to side plank:

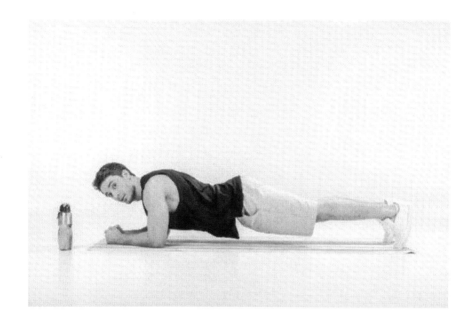

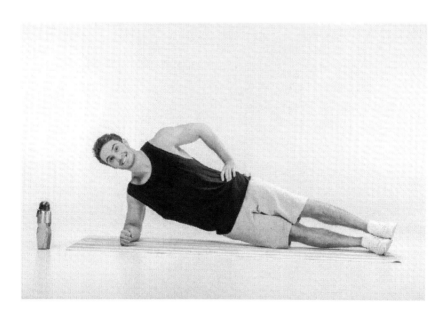

How:

1. Start in pushup position with your back straight and body forming a straight diagonal line from head to shoulders
2. Perform a pushup
3. As you rise back up from the pushup, shift your weight onto your left arm and roll onto your left forearm/elbow
4. Rotate your body to the left until your right side is facing the ceiling. Hold this position for several seconds, then roll back onto both arms and return to the starting pushup position
5. Repeat but instead roll onto your right side.
6. Continue repeating for indicated set

Breathing:

Inhale as you lower into the pushup, exhale as you rise up into the plank and hold your breath during the plank.

Best Practices:

- It's very important to keep your back perfectly straight through out the whole exercise. It's better to get the form right so reduce the number of reps at first if you're struggling with the form.

Try: 10 reps, 3 sets. Increase to 20 reps per set as you improve.

Primary Muscle Group: Obliques, core, full body

4). Oblique Throwdown:

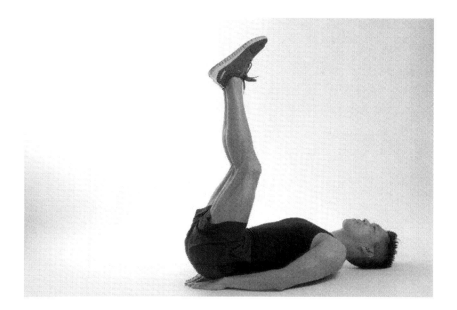

How:

1. Start by lying face up, back on the floor, keep your leg straight and arms underneath your hips. Your legs should be raised perpendicular to the floor keeping them as straight as possible.
2. Lower your legs keeping your feet together until they almost touch the floor, then kick them back up as high as you can without bending your knees.
3. Continue repeating for the duration of the set.

Breathing:

- Breathe in as you lift your legs.
- Breathe out as you lower your legs.

Best Practices:

- Keep the motion controlled and precise—don't rely on momentum to swing your legs up and down

For Added Emphasis: use an exercise partner and have them stand hedind your head. When your legs go up, have them grab your feet and push them back down to the ground as hard as they can. This will add resistance and make it a more effective exercise.

Try:

- Do 2 to 3 sets of 8 to 12 repetitions.

Primary Muscles: Abs, obliques

Secondary Muscles: Lower Back, Hip Flexor, Thighs

---

5). Side Plank Up and Downs:

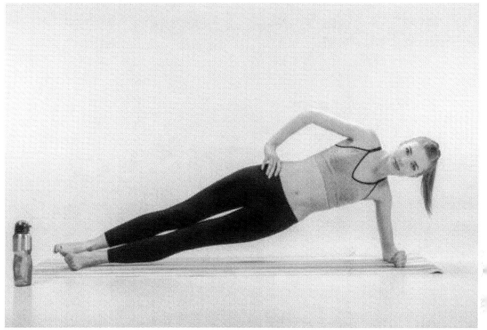

How:

1. Follow the same steps for the side plank (listed earlier in this section).
2. When you are in the plank position, rather than holding your body perfectly straight, allow your mid section to droop towards the floor.
3. Since you are propped up on your elbow, allow your hip closest to the floor to droop, and then push your midsection back up flexing your oblique muscles.
4. Push your hip back up until your body is in a perfectly straight diagonal line again (from your head to your toes). And hold for 3-5 seconds
5. Repeat

Breathing:

Inhale as you allow your body to droop, exhale as you push your hip back up to start position.

Best Practices:

When you rock your hip back up to start position, really focus on clenching your oblique muscles on your side that's facing the ceiling. Use your obliques to pull your body back up rather than momentum.

Try: 60 seconds continuous, do 4 sets.

Primary Muscle Group: Obliques

Section 4: Core Exercises

1). Plank

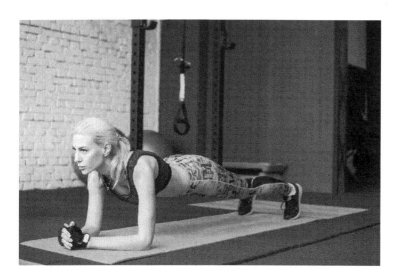

How:

1. Lay flat on your stomach on a carpeted floor or mat.
2. Push your body up on your elbows and put your feet together balancing on the balls of your feet or your toes if you're wearing shoes.

3. Keep your back a straight diagonal line from your shoulders to your feet.
4. Clench your core and tighten your abs and hold for the duration of the set.

Breathing:

This is a continuous burn, so breath deeply and slowly throughout the exercise.

Best Practices:

- It's very important to keep your back as straight as possible. Your body will naturally want to droop towards the floor, but don't let it.
- Lock your hands/arms together in front of you as you're propped on your elbows for extra support and to anchor yourself.

For Added Emphasis:

You can either increase the plank time, or put some sort of weight on your back (such as a heavy book or dictionary).

Try: 60 Seconds plank, 30 seconds rest. Do 3 sets. As you improve, increase your plant time to 2 minutes (decrease the number of sets if necessary).

Primary Muscle: Core

Secondary: Full Body

2). Sit Ups:

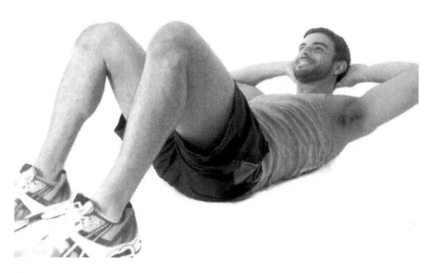

How:

1. Lie flat on your back on a carpeted floor or a mat.
2. Bend your knees and plant your feet flat on the ground about a foot from your butt.
3. Place your hands behind your head and lock your fingers bending your elbows.
4. Raise your upper back and head off the ground bringing your upper body towards your knees.
5. Lower upper body back towards the floor, but don't allow your shoulders to touch the ground.
6. Repeat

Breathing:

Exhale as you raise your upper body, inhale as you lower it towards the floor.

Best Practices:

Try to pull yourself up with your abs. Focus on tightening them as much as possible. You do not need a huge range of motion, its better to have a smaller range of motion and focus on really pulling with your abs.

For Added Emphasis:

Elevate your feet onto a chair, Or try holding a dumbbell carefully on your chest while performing the situps (even 5 pounds will greatly increase the difficulty)

Try: Set 1: 50 situps, Set 2: 40 Situps, Set 3: 30 Situps, Set 4: 20 Situps, Set 5: 10 situps.

Primary Muscle Group: Core, Abs

3). Sit up and Twist:

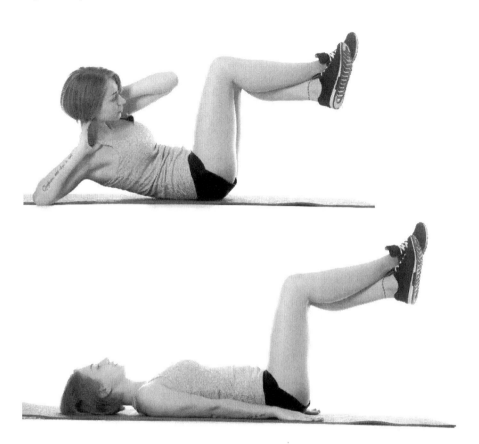

How:

1. Follow the same steps you used for the situps.
2. When you raise your upper body towards your knees rotate your body to the left so your right elbow points towards your left knee.
3. Return to start position, then repeat rotating to the right so that your left elbow points towards your right knee.

Breathing:

Exhale as you sit up, inhale as you lower your back to the start position.

Best Practices: try to push yourself to rotate as far as you possibly can to the right or left and try to pull with your abs instead of using momentum to rock your body up and down.

Try: *25 situps, 4 sets.*

Primary Muscle: Core, Abs

4). Sit ups with legs raised:

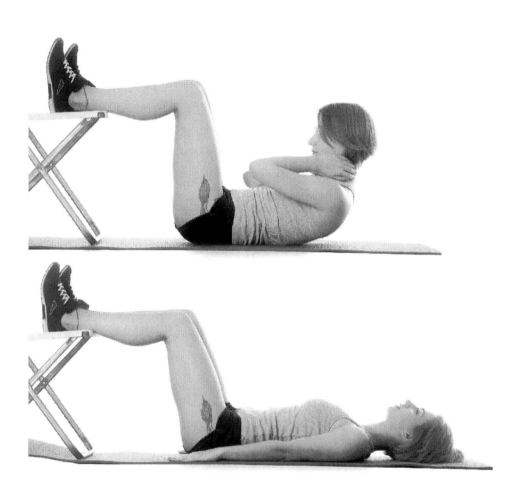

How:

1. Follow the same steps as the "Sit-up" described earlier in this section.
2. Instead of planting your feet on the floor, bend your knees and place your feet on the seat of a chair. Your legs should form a 90 degree angle (shins parallel to the floor).
3. Perform the sit-up as described previously.

Breathing: Exhale as you sit up, inhale as you lower back to the starting position.

For Added Emphasis:

You can try the twist variation with your feet elevated as well (follow the instructions for the "Sit-Up and Twist" exercise.

Try: *40 situps per set, 3 sets*

Primary Muscle: Core, Abs

---

5). Wall Plank:

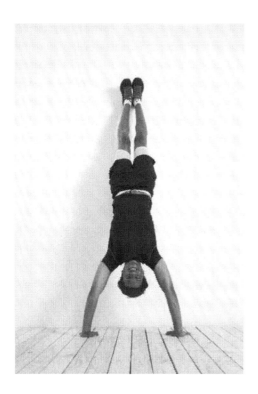

How:

1. Set your hands on the floor and keeping shoulders-width apart.
2. Keep hands slightly wider and head should be in the forward position of your hands.
3. Push yourself up the wall with your back facing the wall and raise yourself up on your hands so you're basically doing a hand stand with the backs of your heels resting against the wall
4. Once your head & hands are in position Hold this posture for 60 seconds, but don't forget to breathe.

5. Slowly return by shifting your weight on the right hand and take one leg into the wall.
6. Then lower the other leg safely to the ground.

Breathing:

- Take continuous deep breaths

Best Practices:

- Keeps your back facing the wall throughout the exercise and try to keep your body in a straight line.
- Your fingers should be pointing straight and keep elbows locked in all the way.
- If the form is too hard don't attempt it. You could hurt yourself.

Try:

- 30 seconds plank, 30 seconds rest, 3 sets.

Primary Muscles: Abs

Secondary Muscles: Triceps, Hip flexors, Obliques, Claves

6). Russian Twist

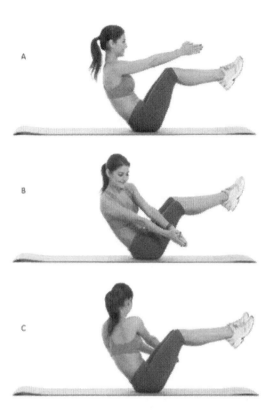

How:

1. Sit on the ground (carpet or a yoga mat) with your feet stretched in front of you.
2. Kick your feet out in front of you and raise them off the ground several inches (keep your feet together) and bend at the knee slightly)
3. Rock back onto your lower back slightly keeping your back and shoulders elevated.
4. Clasp your hands together in your lap (so you are only balancing on your butt and lower back).

5. Rotate your body to the left as you simultaneously move your clasped hands to your side and touch the ground by your left hip.
6. Rotate back front and center and then repeat rotating this time to the right and touching your clasped hands to the ground next to your right hip.
7. Repeat for the duration of the set.

Breathing:

This is a continuous burn so it may be difficult to effectively coordinate your breathing. You may just want to take measured slow, deep breaths. Or you can try exhaling as you twist and inhaling as you return to center.

Best Practices: If you cannot stay balanced on your butt and lower back, this exercise wont be effective. If you have trouble keeping your balance, try with your feet elevated on a stool or low chair. Once you've mastered that, take the chair away and try again.

For Added Emphasis:

Hold a medicine ball instead of clasping your hands together. Take a medicine ball (between 5-10 lbs) in both hands and perform the exercise touching it to the ground on either side as you twist.

Try: *30 Seconds Continuous, 30 seconds rest. 3 sets.*

Primary Muscle: Core, Obliques, Abs

Secondary Muscle: Quads

7). Burpee

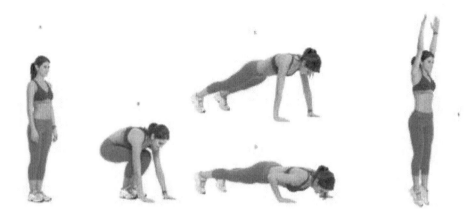

How to:

1. Stand with your feet about shoulder width apart.
2. Quickly drop into a crouching position with your hips back and touch your hands to the ground as pictured.
3. Shifting your weight onto your hands for support, kick your legs back until you're in a pushup position.
4. Then jump your legs back up to the crouching position and spring upward on you feet jumping into the air with your hands stretched upward.
5. When you land back in your start position, repeat the exercise for the indicated number of reps.

Breathing:

Since this is a dynamic exercise, try to just take steady measured breaths throughout.

For Added Emphasis:

At step three, when you're in the pushup position, you can actually perform a pushup to make the exercise more difficult (see the picture).

Primary Muscle Group: Core, full body

8). Bird Dog:

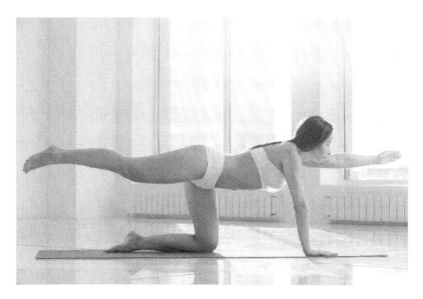

How:

1. Start on your hands and knees on all fours
2. Keep your hands under your shoulders and keeps your knees straightly under your hips.
3. Lift your right arm onward and lift your left leg in a backward position.
4. In this process keep your backs & pelvis firm and still and don't move the pelvis, but keep your whole body in a straight line from head to toe.
5. Just focus on the rib cage and don't sag it towards the floor.
6. This will engage the muscles and stabilize your spine.
7. Go back to the starting position by placing your knee or hands on the ground.
8. Repeat this process on the other side and get a complete one rep.

Breathing:

- Exhale and Inhale at the same time when you lift your right arm and left leg.

Best practices:

- It is good for you to perform better and few bird dogs with excellent form.
- You must do with your strengths and steadily go with the level of workout. If you can only lift arm, then take a time to get expertise.

Try:

- Do 5 to 10 reps on each side.

Primary Muscles: Middle and lower back and abs

Secondary Muscles: Glutes, hip flexors

---

9). Upward Plank:

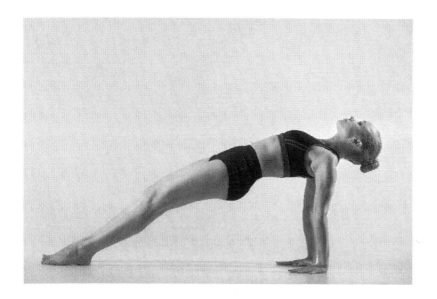

How:

1. Start in pictured pose by keeping your hands on the floor some inches behind your hips. (Palms down, body facing the ceiling)
2. Keep your fingers in a forward position, and then bend your knees by placing your feet on the floor.
3. Inhale and lift your hips off the mat.
4. Keep in this position for 30 seconds and go back to the Dandasana (start) pose with an exhalation.

Breathing:

- Inhale as you raise your hips and exhale as you back down to the Dandasana.

Best practices:

- If you have a neck or wrist injury, so must do this pose with care.

- If it looks too difficult then do practice with the tabletop that builds strength & steadiness.
- Practicing upward plank can boost and support your mind & body, but you need to practice correctly.

Try:

- Hold the pose for 5 to 10 breaths

Primary Muscles: Arm, Leg & Wrist, core

Secondary Muscles: Front ankle, Shoulder, Thorax

10). Reverse Crunch:

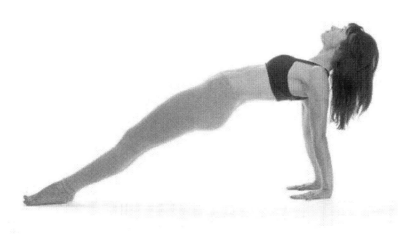

How:

1. Lie on the floor and keep your hands by your sides.
2. Keep your legs straight in front of you and raise your knees at a 90-degree angle.
3. Your thighs and calves should be parallel to the floor.
4. Inhale and lift your hips and bring your legs towards your torso.
5. Keep your knees towards your face and tilt your feet towards the sky.
6. Exhale and back to your starting position, but never drop your legs quickly.

Breathing:

- Exhale when you lift your legs off and inhale as you slowly come to starting position.

Best practices:

- It strengthens your abs and enhances core and lower back stability.

- If you are beginner then slowly concentrate on proper form and it is best for beginners to keep their knees close to the body.

Try:

- You can do 15 to 20 reps and Complete 3 to 5 sets. But don't get worried if you can't do many reps.

Primary Muscles: Abs

Secondary muscles: Abs

11). Plank Raised leg

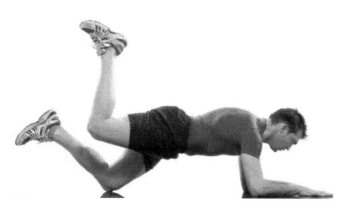

How:

1. This is a variation of the regular plank (see the page on the plank exercise earlier in this section).
2. Instead of planting your feet on the ground, elevate them on a low chair or stool so that your body forms a straight line parallel to the ground. You will still be propped up on your elbows.
3. Tighten your core and flex your abs as you hold the position for the duration of the set.

Breathing:

This is a continuous burn, so take measured consistent breaths throughout the exercise.

Best Practices:

Try to keep your back as straight as possible (even arch it out slightly if necessary to avoid drooping.

For Added Emphasis:

Elevate your feet on a higher stool or chair so your body is slanting downward (your feet are higher than the rest of your body). This is basically a decline plank and will be more difficult.

Try: *45 seconds plank, 30 seconds rest. 3 sets.*

Primary Muscle: Core

Secondary: Full Body

12). Crunch:

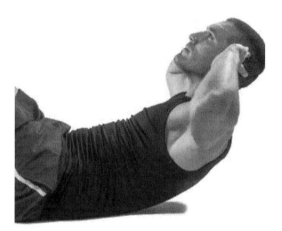

How:

1. Lie on the floor on your back and keep your feet flat on the floor.
2. Place your hands firmly on both sides of the head and keep your elbows out.
3. Slowly pushing down your back to the floor and isolate abdominal muscles (push and pull with your abs)

4. Now start to roll your shoulders to the ground.
5. Your shoulders should be off to the ground about 3 to 4 inches, but keep your lower back flat on the floor. Make sure let your abs works slowly and in a controlled manner.

Breathing:

- You should breathe out while exerting yourself and breathe in when you end the movement

Best practices:

- If you are a beginner and pain problem in your lower back, then you can use an abdominal crunch machine.
- This will never put extra pressure on your back and it strengthens your abdominal core.

Try:

- Do 30 to 50 repetitions and must complete 3 to 5 sets.

Primary muscles: Rectus Abdominus

Secondary muscles: Transverse Abdominus, Internal and External Oblique's

13). Dead Bug:

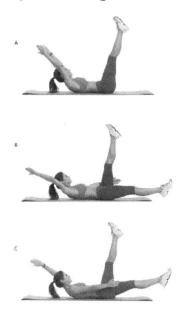

How:

1. Lie down and keep your back flat on the floor.
2. Keep your hands and legs in front of you pointing towards the ceiling.
3. Bring your right leg up and lower your left arm at the same time.
4. Come back to starting position and repeat the same process with opposite arms & legs.
5. Continue switching sides for the sets.

Breathing:

- Exhale as you lower your leg and lift your arm
- Inhale when you come back to starting position and switch sides.

Best practices:

- You have to careful while doing dead bug and keep your back flat on the floor as it will otherwise place too much pressure on your back.
- The dead bug is a great core move that enhances core strength, organization, stability, and flexibility.

Try:

- Do 8 to 12 repetitions which complete approximately 4 sets on each side.

Primary Muscles: Abs

Secondary Muscles: Core

14). Plank Jack:

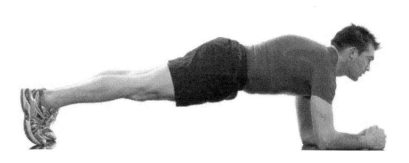

How:

1. Start with your toes and forearms on the floor and form your body into a straight line by keeping your feet together and back straight.
2. Hop slightly with your toes and extend your legs as far as you can.
3. Jump again slightly and bring your feet back together. (almost like a laying down jumping jack)
4. Repeat for indicated number of reps.

Breathing:

- Throughout the exercise process maintain slow and steady breathing pattern.

Best practices:

- This exercise requires core strength, shoulder and muscular stability & endurance.
- You should keep your spine stable and never drop your hips towards the ground.
- But if you are beginner then start with these two exercises, jumping jacks & regular planks and practiced properly.

Try:

- You can do plank jacks continuously for 30 seconds to 1 minute per set. Complete 3 sets

Primary Muscles: Core

Secondary Muscles: Shoulders, lower body

15). Rolling Side Plank:

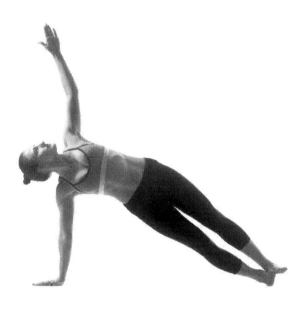

How:

1. Start in plank position and lie on your right side keeping your feet together.
2. Keep your forearms on the ground, lift your whole body off to the ground and keep your ankles & shoulders in a straight line.
3. Hold in the side plank position flexing your oblique muscles.
4. Maintain your balance and lower your body into the front plank position. (Lowering yourself into a

pushup or front plank positions before switching sides)

5. Put your weight on both elbows and forearms and keep your body in a straight line.
6. Change the side plank to the other side and manage your body in a straight line from shoulders to ankles.

Breathing:

- You must keep a steady breathing pattern throughout this workout.

Best Practices:

- Firstly, you should be able to do side plank or traditional plank individually before attempting this exercise.
- The rolling side plank will reduce the back pain and give you a strong core.

Try:

- Perform the one side plank for 60 seconds and don't let your hips or back sag during the process. Then roll to the other side 60 seconds. Then take a 60 second break. Try to work your way up to 3 sets of this.

Primary Muscles: Abs, Obliques

Secondary muscles: Shoulders, Quads, Glutes and lower back

16). Box Jump:

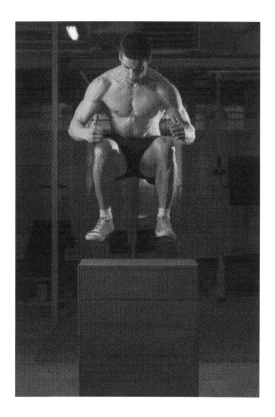

How:

1. Stand in front of the box or some kind of sturdy raised object. Keep your hands by your sides and legs slightly bent.
2. Keep yourself in crouching jumping position and bend your knees & hips.
3. Explosively jump forward from the bent position by swinging your arms.
4. Land on the box lightly also in the crouch position
5. Immediately and jump back & return to starting position.

6. Repeat this sequence.

Breathing:

- Inhale when you bend and start to box jump.
- Exhale as you jump back to the starting position.

Best practices:

- Accuracy and balance are two important parts for the proper execution of the best box jump
- It's better to start with a low box or step until that becomes easy for you before going for something a little higher
- Avoid using an unstable box as it may increase injury risk.

Try:

- 2 to 3 sets of 5-8 reps

Primary Muscles: Quadriceps

Secondary Muscles: Calves, Hamstrings

Section 5: Chest Exercises

1). Wide arm Pushups:

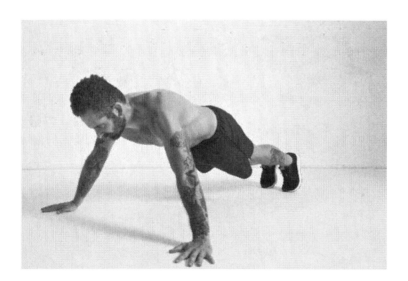

How:

1. Lay on your stomach on a matt or carpeted area.
2. Get into pushup position (back straight feet planted together on the floor elevated onto your hands.
3. Space your hands widely in front of you (almost elbow width) so your elbows make 90 degree angles.
4. Perform the pushup.
5. Repeat for the indicated number of reps.

Breathing:

Inhale as you lower your body, exhale as you raise it back up to start position.

Best Practices:

- Keep your back straight (don't let it droop)
- Try to go as low as possible without compromising your form.

Try:

15 pushups, 4 sets. Increase the number every time (even if it's only 1 more pushup per set).

Primary Muscle: Chest

Secondary: Back, Shoulders, Full Body

2). Narrow Grip Pushups:

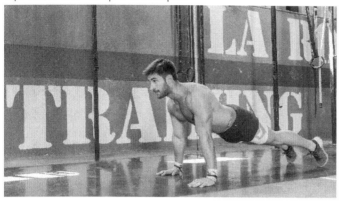

How:

1. Follow the same instructions listed in the previous exercise, but instead of holding a wide grip, move your hands very close together until they're only a few inches apart.
2. Keep your arms straight, and bend at the elbow when performing the exercise
3. Lower your body as far as you can and then push yourself back up to the start position keeping your back as straight as possible.

Breathing: Inhale as you lower, exhale as you raise.

Best Practices: Squeeze your pecs as you perform the exercise (especially when pushing yourself back up) and keep your back straight.

Try:*15 pushups, 4 sets. Increase the number of pushups per set as you improve.*

Primary Muscle: Chest, Core, Triceps

Secondary: Shoulders, Full Body

3). Single Arm Pushups:

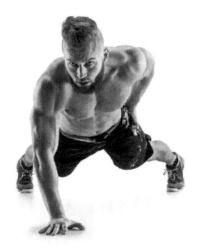

How:

1. Get into regular pushup position.
2. Once you've achieved a comfortable balance, pull one of your hands off the floor and tuck it behind your back or hold it next to your side.
3. Perform the pushup in normal form using only one arm.
4. Repeat for recommended number of reps and then switch sides.

Breathing: Inhale when you're going down, exhale when you're pushing yourself back up.

Best Practices: You may want to spread your feet wider apart than normal to help you keep your balance.

Try: *5 reps each arm, repeat 3 times or until failure.*

Primary Muscle: Chest, Triceps, Arms

4). Dumbell Pushup Pulls:

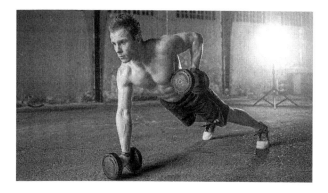

*In order to perform this exercise, you will need dumbbells of some type. The heavier the weight, the more difficult the exercise

How:

1. Place two dumbbells on the ground about shoulder-width apart.
2. Get into normal pushup position but instead of placing your hands flat on the floor, grip the dumbbells with each hand. The dumbells should be laid length-wise so that when you grip them, your palms are facing each other.
3. Perform the pushup lowering yourself as far as you can go.
4. When you return to start position, raise the dumbbell in your right hand as far up as you can (bending at the elbow) until the dumbbell touches your chest, then return it to the ground.
5. Repeat with another pushup, and then raise the left dumbbell.
6. Repeat alternating for the duration of the set.

Breathing:

Inhale as you lower your body, and then slowly start to exhale as you raise back up to start position, and continue to exhale as you raise the dumbbell.

For Added Emphasis: Instead of stopping when you raise the dumbbell to your chest, rotate your body away from the dumbbell and continue raising it to the sky until your arm is straight

Try:*30 Seconds, continuous, 30 seconds rest. Do 3 sets. Increase either the weight of the dumbbells or the time per set (or both) as you improve.*

Primary Muscle: Chest

Secondary: Back, Arms, Full Body

5). Decline Pushups:

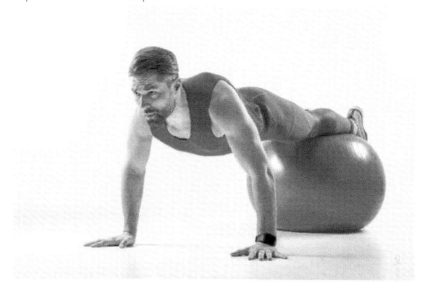

How:

1. Get into pushup position, but instead of planting your legs flat on the ground, elevate them onto the seat of a chair. If the chair is not high enough, place some large books on the chair beneath your feet.
2. Your body should be pointing downward in a diagonal line (feet highest, head lowest)
3. Perform the pushups at a decline for the indicated number of reps.

Breathing: Inhale as you lower your body, exhale as you push up.

Best Practices: The higher your legs are elevated the more effective (and more difficult) the exercise. Make sure to keep your back straight the whole time.

Try: *15 pushups, 5 sets. Increase the number of reps and/or sets as you improve.*

Primary Muscle: Upper Chest

Secondary: Back, Shoulders, Full Body

---

6). Chest Dips (on a counter or two chairs):

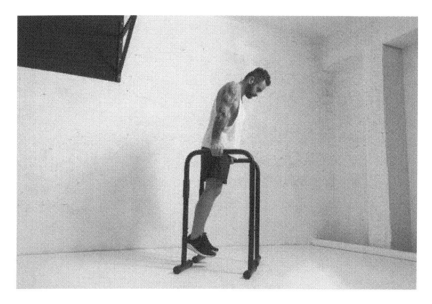

This exercise can be difficult to perform at home, so only do it if you feel comfortable with it

How:

1. Locate a space between two kitchen counters that is 2-3 ft wide.
2. Place your hands on the edge of the two counters with your body in between them and push yourself up until your arms are straight.
3. Bend your legs behind you and lock your feet together.
4. Slowly lower your body downwards and forward simultaneously as far as you can without failing. (try to go so far that your elbows form a 90 degree angle)
5. Then push yourself back up to start position. Repeat for the indicated number of reps.

Breathing:

Inhale as you lower your body, exhale as you push yourself back up.

Best Practices:

- If you don't push yourself forward when you're lowering your body, you wont be working your chest. You will almost be lowering your self at a downward diagonal angle. If you go straight up and down, that will work only your triceps (which is still good, but not what we're going for here).
- If you don't have kitchen counters that will work, some people perform this exercise between two chairs holding the chair backs. I do not recommend this unless you feel your chairs are sturdy enough (you don't want them to tip because you could injure yourself).

Try: *10 dips, 3 sets. Increase the number of dips per set as you improve.*

Primary Muscle: Chest, Triceps

7). Incline Pushups:

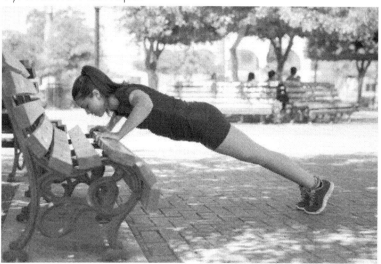

How:

1. Find a high step, or a stool or a low chair and lower yourself into pushup position with your hands on the elevated surface.
2. Keep your feet together and firmly planted on the ground with your back straight.
3. Your body should be forming a diagonal line upwards (feet lowest, head highest).
4. Perform the pushups for the indicated number of reps.

Breathing: Inhale as you lower your body, exhale as you push up.

Best Practices: Make sure the elevated surface you choose is not too tall. You want it to be tall enough to make a difference, but not so tall that you're not doing any work

Try: 20 pushups, 4 sets.

Primary Muscle: Chest, Back

Secondary: Shoulders, Arms, Full Body

8). Pushup Hold

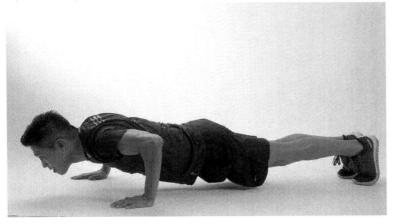

How to:

1. Perform the pushup as described in any of the earlier pushup exercises in this book.
2. When pushing back up to the start position, hold in the start position tightening your core. Hold for 10 seconds
3. Repeat for indicated number of reps

Breathing:

Since you are doing short planks throughout the exercise, just focus on taking long deep breaths throughout.

Best Practices: when you return to start position to hold, do not lock your elbows, keep your arms slightly bent to force a strain.

Try: *10 pushups, 3 sets.*

Primary Muscle: Core, Chest

9). Chest Squeeze Rotation

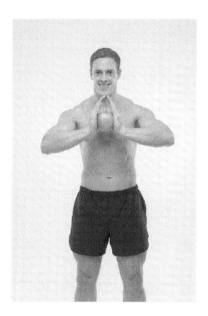

How to:

1. Stand up straight with feet shoulder width apart.
2. Take a heavy book (such as a dictionary) and hold it like a pancake with your hands spread and flat gripping the front and back cover. (your palms should be facing each other almost as if you're praying with a book between your hands).
3. Hold it out in front of you and start to rotate the book in a circle keeping a tight grip and pushing your hands as hard together as possible squeezing your chest muscles.
4. Rotate in circles (about the extent of comfortable arm's reach) for the duration of the set. (the circle should be outward, circling away from your body).

Breathing:

Take slow, measured breaths throughout.

Best Practices:

Really focus on squeezing your palms together as tightly as you can (almost as if you're trying to push through the book) and drive the force from your chest muscles. Squeeze your pecs together and hold.

For Added Emphasis:

Perform a set clockwise, and then immediately perform one counterclockwise without resting between them.

Try: *30 seconds continuous, 30 seconds rest. (4 sets)*

Primary Muscle: Chest

Secondary: Arms

10). Pullups:

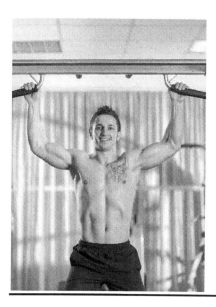

How:

1. Grasp the bar with your hands shoulder-width apart and arm completely extended.
2. Now pull up towards the bar turning your hands and pull steadily until your chin touches the bar.
3. Keep in this position for 1 or 2 seconds and then slowly lower yourself back down until your arms are extended again.
4. Now go back to the starting position and do the above process again.

Breathing:

- Exhale as you start to perform pull-up
- Inhale while you are coming down

Best practice:

- Try to pull with your chest and back muscles and don't use momentum to swing your body up and down
- If the bar is too low so that your feet are touching the ground, touch your feet behind you so that you're not using your feet or legs for support.

Try:

- Perform 20 to 28 reps in however many sets it takes you

Primary Muscles: Biceps, Latissimus Dorsi

Secondary Muscles: Upper back muscles, Forearm muscles, Abdominal

Section 6: Back Exercises:

1). Dumbell Lat Raise

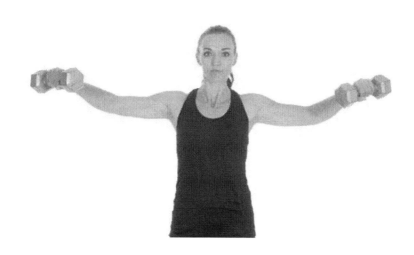

How:

1. Stand up straight and grab a pair of dumbbells.
2. Grip the dumbells overhand, palms facing in.
3. Lift your arms at your sides keeping your arms straight with the elbows just slightly bent.

4. Once your arms form 90 degree angles and are parallel to the ground, hold the position for a moment, then lower them back down.

5. Repeat

Breathing:

- Exhale when you're raising your arms, inhale when you're lowering them.

Best practices:

- Do not swing your arms or use momentum—use your lats to really pull the weight up and lower it very slowly and in a very controlled movement.

Try:

- Do 3 sets of 8 to 12 repetitions

Primary Muscles: Lats, Middle Deltoid (Shoulders)

Secondary Muscles: Arms, upper back, shoulders, chest

2). Chin ups:

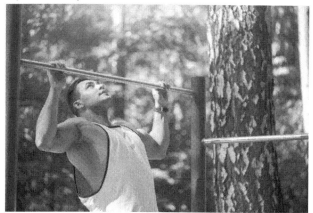

How:

1. Grasp the bar overhand, gripping about shoulder width apart or wider.
2. Brace your Abs and squeeze your glutes by taking deep breaths.
3. Pull yourself up keeping your chin upward the level of the bar.
4. After that, slowly lower back to starting position and repeat again.

Breathing:

- Inhale when you pull yourself upward.
- Exhale when you complete the exercise

Best practice:

- Concentrate on accurate moves during exercise and slowly return to the starting point.

Try: 20 reps in as many sets as it takes.

Primary Muscles: Biceps, Latissimus Dorsi

Secondary Muscles: Abdominals, upper back muscles, delts

4). Good Mornings:

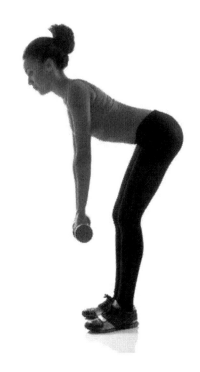

How to do:

1. Stand tall with your feet flat toes pointing slightly outwards about shoulder-width apart
2. Put your hands behind your head, bending elbows
3. Bend at the waist until your torso is parallel to the ground keeping your legs straight.
4. Exhale and return to the starting position and repeat.

Breathing:

- Inhale as you lower your chest

- Exhale as you repeat the exercise from starting position

Best practices:

- Arch your back throughout this exercise to make sure to target your lower back
- Really push with your lower back muscles instead of just snapping your body back up

For Added Emphasis:

Hold dumbells by your sides (as pictured) instead of keeping your hands behind your head.

Try:

- Do 3 sets of 20 reps

Primary Muscles: Hamstrings

Secondary Muscles: Lower back, calves, Glutes

5). Superman:

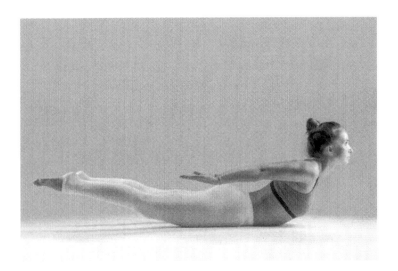

How:

1. Lie on the ground on your belly and keep your arms & legs completely extended. Arms should be at your sides palms facing the ceiling.
2. Raise your arms & legs simultaneously off the floor and hold on this position for several seconds.
3. Go back to the starting position and repeat the process.

Breathing:

- Inhale as you lift your arms & legs off the floor.
- Exhale when you down the arms or legs and keep on the next rep.

Best practice:

- The Superman exercise helps to strengthen your core by using middle and lower back.

- This exercise is all about flexinf your core. When you're holding the superman position, flex your abs and tighten your body to really feel the burn.

Try:

- You set your superman exercise routine by adding 2 to 3 sets of 10 to 16 repetitions.

Primary Muscles: Lower back, Middle back

Secondary Muscles: Abs

6). Scapular Pushup:

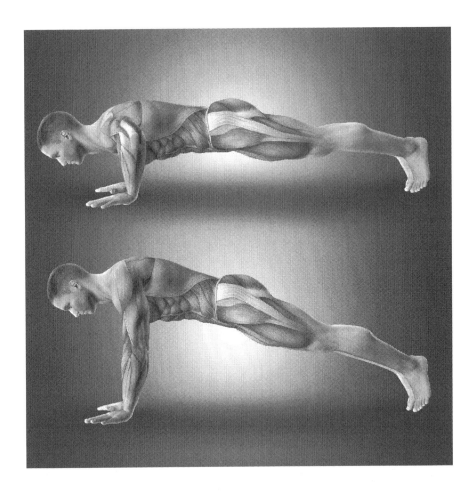

How to do:

1. Start in the plank position, placing your hands straight beneath the shoulders.
2. Keep your toes on the ground and keep your body in a straight line.

3. Tighten your Abs and perform the pushup not allowing your back to arch.
4. Extend your arms and pinch your shoulder blades together.
5. Keep in this position for 5 seconds, then release and go back to the plank position.

Breathing:

- Breathe in when you push yourself forward
- Breathe out when you push back

Best practice:

- Keeping your back from bowing out is key.
- When you've lowered yourself into the pushup, squeeze your shoulder blades together as tightly as possible.

Try:

- 3 sets of 15 to 20 repetitions.

Primary Muscles: Back, Torso

Secondary Muscles: Abs, Shoulders, Arms

Section 7: TRICEP Exercises

1). Tricep Dips

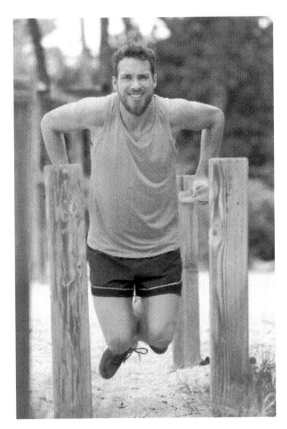

See exercise earlier in this book for chest dips

How:

1. Follow the same instructions for the chest dips listed in an earlier section, but instead of dipping forward, just dip straight up and down
2. You will have to lean forward slightly, but just focus on pushing yourself up with your triceps.
3. Go as far down as you can until your arms form 90 degree angles but keep your shoulders open and wide to avoid using them.

Breathing:

Inhale as you lower yourself, exhale as you raise up

Best Practices;

Just as with chest dips, you can use two kitchen counters that are a suitable distance apart, or try to use two chair backs at your own risk. If you feel the strain heavily in your shoulders, try keeping your shoulders back and pushing your chest out while you perform the exercise.

Try: 10 dips, 4 sets (increase the number of dips per set as you improve)

Primary Muscle: Triceps

Secondary: Shoulders, Chest

2). Diamond Pushups:

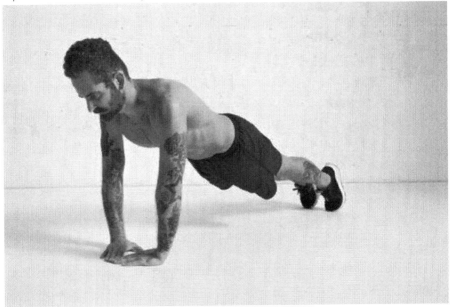

How:

1. Reference the "Narrow Grip Pushups" exercise which is in the "Chest" section of this book.
2. Instead of simply holding your hands close together, push your palms all the way together and extend your thumbs so they're touching each other.
3. Your hands should form a diamond or triangle between your forefingers and thumbs.
4. Repeat for the indicated number of reps.

Breathing: inhale when you're going down, exhale when you're coming back up.

Primary Muscle: Triceps, Chest

Secondary: Shoulders, Back

3). Tricep Pushups:

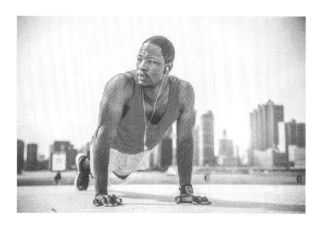

How:

1. Get into pushup position but keep your hands at a narrow stance—shoulder width apart.
2. Perform the pushup keeping your elbows in and arms narrow so you're pushing and pulling with your triceps.
3. Using your pectoral muscles & biceps push your body to return to the starting position.
4. Pause for 1 second at this position and repeat the exercise set again (Do 1-second pause, 1-second push and 1 second down count)

Breathing:

- Inhale as you push yourself down
- Exhale as you push yourself back

Best practices:

- Your elbows will want to go out, but concentrate on keeping them in so you're really using your triceps for this exercise.

Try:

- 3-4 sets of 10-15

Primary Muscles: Triceps, Chest

Secondary Muscles: Abs, Shoulders, Arms

4) Narrow Grip Incline Pushup

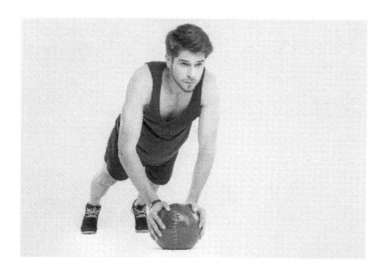

How to:

1. Take a perfect pushup position with your hands on a medicine ball. Or even just flat on the ground in front of you about 3-5 inches apart.
2. Place the medicine ball under your torso.
3. Keep your hand's thumbs and fingers together.
4. Support your core by keeping your arms completely extended.
5. Keep your elbows close to your body and slowly perform the pushup
6. Pause for a second and push yourself back to the starting position.

Breathing:

- Inhale when you come down towards the ball.
- Exhale when you lift your body to go back to the starting position.

Best practices:

- Don't try it on the medicine ball until you can accurately perform narrow grip pushups.

Try:

- Do 3 sets of 10 to 15 reps

Primary Muscles: Triceps

Secondary Muscles: Biceps, Delts, Pectorals

5). Exercise Band Pulldown

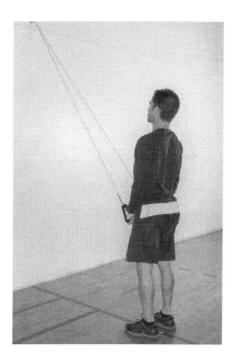

How to do:

- Loop an exercise band around something about eye level height that is sturdy and wont break so that the ends of the band are hanging about shoulder level
- Stand straight with legs and slightly bent at your knees.
- Keep your back straight and your arms at shoulder height.
- Grasp the band in each hand and keeping your elbows at your sides, pull the band down without moving the top half of your arms. Only use your forearms and hands

- Slowly raise your arms as you release the band back to starting position

Breathing:

- Breathe out when you pull down
- Breathe in as you go back to starting point.

Best practice:

- Keep your elbows and shoulders in and perfectly still
- If you're not feeling it isolated in your triceps, move around until you feel it there

Try:

- Complete 3 sets of 25 reps

Primary Muscles: Triceps, Upper back, lats

Secondary Muscles: Shoulders, biceps

Section8: Bicep Exercises

1). Band Curl:

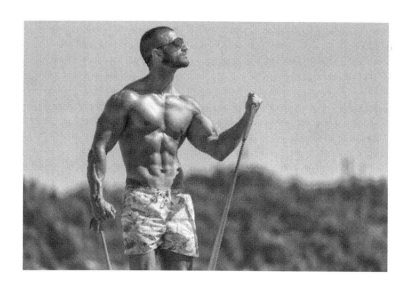

How:

1. Loop the band beneath your feet about hip-width apart and grab each band handle with a palm-up grip.

2. Stand tall and keep your lower back straight, elbows slightly bent to your sides, abs tight.
3. Curl the band upwards with your left arm keeping your elbows straight and flexing your biceps.
4. Once you've curled all the way up, really squeeze your biceps and hold for a moment.
5. Then lower your arm releasing the tension
6. Repeat with your right arm and continue alternating every time

Breathing:

- Exhale when you curl the band toward your torso.
- Inhale when you slowly come back to the starting position.

Best Practices:

- During this workout never let your elbows move forward & back, but keep elbows immobile at your sides.

Try:

- Do 10 to 12 reps per arm, 3 sets.

Primary Muscles: Biceps

Secondary Muscles: Forearms

2). Inverted Row:

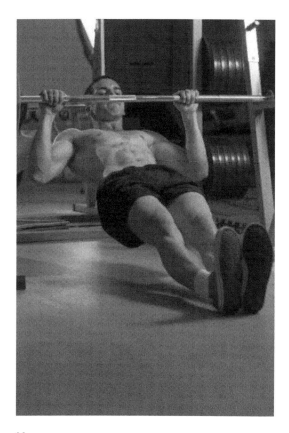

How:

1. For this you will need to find something sturdy that is about waist level off the ground
2. Lie on the ground below the bar (or whatever you're using) and lie flat on your back. Grab the bar underhanded palms facing away from you and legs extended in front of you feet together
3. Pull yourself up towards the bar until your nose is almost touching it.
4. Slowly lower yourself back down but don't let your back touch the ground again until the set is completed

Breathing:

Exhale as you're pulling yourself towards the bar, inhale as you're lowering yourself back down.

Best Practices:

- keep your back as straight as possible and don't bend at the waist or knees. Try to keep your body in a perfectly straight line at all times.

Try: 25 reps, 4 sets

Primary Muscle Group: Biceps, triceps, Shoulders, Upper Body, Lats

3). Towel Chinups:

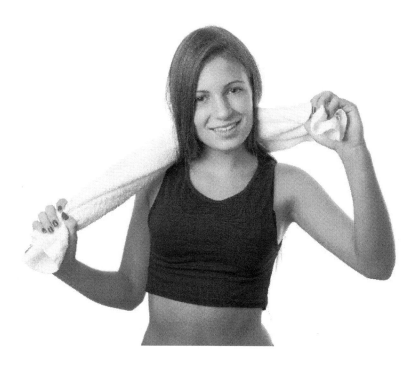

How:

1. Wrap two smaller towels over the chin up bar at shoulders-width apart.
2. Grab the towels in each hand and keep your body in a hand down position, arms extended
3. Lift your feet off the ground and pull yourself up as high as possible
4. Slowly lower your body to the starting point and repeat.

Breathing:

- exhale as you pull up
- inhale as lower yourself back to the floor.

Best Practices:

- You can do this with one towel, but remember to use a good quality towel, which can hold your weight easily.

Try: Do 8 to 12 repetitions.

Primary Muscles: Biceps, Middle back, Lats

Secondary Muscles: Forearms, Biceps

4). Plank Ups:

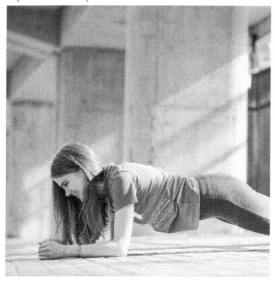

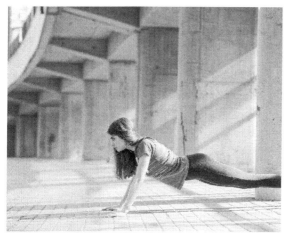

How:

1. Start to the plank position and keep your hands straight under your shoulders, resting on your elbows back straight.
2. Your toes should touch the floor. Squeeze your glutes to stabilize your body.

3. Keep your legs and knees on moving position and your hands should remain in a line.
4. Hold the plank position for 15-20 seconds, then raise up onto your palms, fully extending your arms and flex your core. Hold that position for 10 seconds and then return back onto your elbows for the plank position
5. Continue repeating for indicated set

Breathing:

- Take continuous measured breaths throughout

Best practices:

- Throughout the exercise, keep your spine, head, and neck in a straight line.
- If you are beginner first practice elbow planks and strengthen your core.

Try:

- Do this exercise continuously for 2 minutes, then take a 30 second rest. Do 2-3 sets.

Primary Muscles: Arms, Core

Secondary Muscles: Wrists, Shoulders, Glutes

5). Towel Bicep Curls:

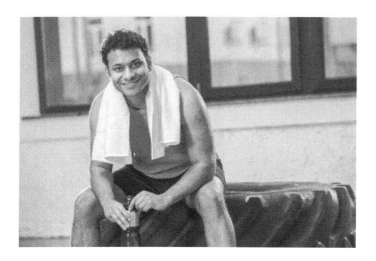

How:

1. Start to standing against the wall and a rolled-up large towel on the floor.
2. Keep a towel in front of you and take a step on the center of the towel with your right foot.
3. Slightly bend and take hold of the ends of the towel in each hand. (Starting Position)
4. Straighten back up with your back against the wall, keep your elbows by your sides.
5. Gradually pull your hands towards shoulders and keep your right knee bent.
6. Slightly push down your right foot back against the towel, for resistance
7. Hold at the top of the curl position flexing your biceps and lower your hands slowly to the starting point.
8. Switch legs and continue.

Breathing:

- Exhale as you perform curls.
- Inhale as you lower your hands and switch the arms.

Best Practices:

- Don't arch your back
- If you have trouble visualizing the steps of this exercise, look up an online video of it for a visual aid.

Try:

- Do 8 to 12 reps per leg, 3 sets

Primary Muscles: Biceps

Secondary Muscles: Forearms

Section 9: Shoulder Exercises

1). Exercise Band Shrugs:

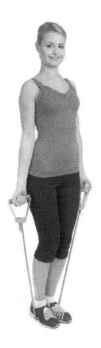

How:

1. Anchor a resistance band below your feet with your feet about shoulder width apart.

2. Grab the two handles of the resistance band—with your arms fully extended at your sides, it should still be slightly resistant
3. Raise your shoulders up at the same time pinching your shoulder blades, but keep your arms completely straight and pinned to your sides
4. Think of this as a shrugging motion
5. Hold the posture and return to start and repeat.

Breathing:

- Exhale when you lift your shoulders.
- Inhale when you lower your Shoulders.

Best Practices:

- Your arms will want to bend at the elbow, but you have to fight that. You must keep your arms perfectly straight and only move your shoulders or else the exercise wont be effective.

Try: Perform 8 to 12 reps of 3sets.

Primary Muscles: Shoulders, Traps

Secondary Muscles: Forearms

2). Handstand wall pushups

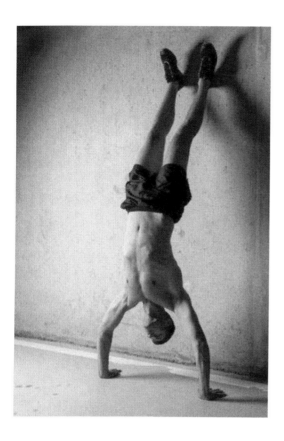

How:

*This is an ambitious exercise, so don't attempt it unless you are confident and know you can do it without injuring yourself

1. Keep your back to the wall bend at the waist.
2. Place your hands in the handstand position on the ground and shoulder-width apart.

3. Keep your arms & legs extended and balance your body.
4. Kick yourself up against the wall and rest your feet on the wall.
5. Keep your arms & legs fully straightened and lower your body until your head approaches the ground.
6. Maintain your balance with the help of the wall and & push-up until arms fully extended again.

Breathing:

- Inhale when you lower yourself for pushups.
- Exhale as you push yourself back to the next push-up.

Best practices:

- It is important to maintain your balance and slowly come down, which is necessary to avoid the risk of injury.
- If you are a beginner, don't do this exercise without any help.
- Select the right distance to the wall and make sure the floor is not slippery.

Try:

- Do 8 to 12 reps of 3 sets.

Primary Muscles: Shoulders

Secondary Muscles: Triceps

3). Pike Pushup:

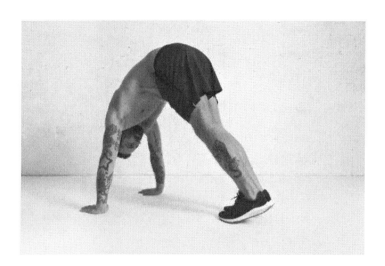

How:

1. Go down on your feet & hands with your palms flat on the ground, shoulder-width apart. Your body should almost form an upside down "U" as you can see in the picture
2. Keep your legs straight and hips up, bend your elbows at 90-degree angle and lowering your upper body towards the floor until your head almost touches the ground.
3. Hold for a second then return to the starting position

Breathing:

- Inhale as you bend your elbows and lower your body to touch the mat.
- Exhale as you push yourself back to the starting point.

Best Practices:

- You will want to keep your legs straight and not engage them much in this exercise. Push and pull with your upper body and only rely on your legs for support and to keep your balance.

Try:

- Complete 3 sets of 15 to 20 reps

Primary Muscles: Shoulders

Secondary Muscles: Upper back, core, Chest, Arms

4). Air Punches:

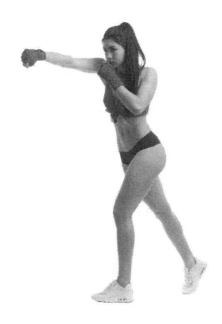

How:

1. Stand up straight with feet shoulder-width apart
2. Move your right foot forward slightly and keep your knees slightly bent.
3. Maintain your position, hands up close to the top of your torso.
4. Start to punch your right hand forward, your elbows locked, arms straight and slightly turn your shoulder

towards the opposite side. If you're punching with your right arm, punch slightly towards the left.

5. The target of your punch should be straight ahead of you at shoulder height.
6. Pull your right arm back and repeat with your left arm.

Breathing:

- Exhale as you push your hand out

Best Practices:

- Air punches improve stamina and help you in losing weight.
- Distribute your weight properly, balancing your body throughout the workout and keep your abs flexed.

Try:

- Do at least 3 sets of 50 repetitions and keep movements swift & smooth but vigorous

Primary Muscles: Shoulders

Secondary Muscles: Triceps, Lats, Biceps

5). Dumbell flies:

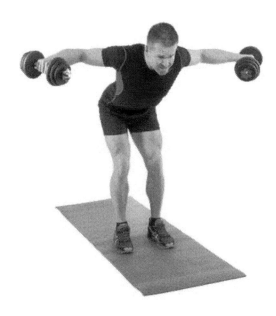

How:

1. Hold a pair of dumbbells with your arms loosely at your sides
2. Bend at the waist about 45 degrees
3. Slowly extend your arms with the dumbells out at your sides keeping your elbows slightly bent.
4. When you've raised them to shoulder height, pause briefly then slowly lower them to the start position
5. repeat

Breathing:

- Exhale as you lift the dumbells
- Inhale as you lower them

Best Practices:

- Keep your elbows in a fixed & stable position and slightly bent throughout the exercise.
- You really want to feel this in your traps so adjust your body until you really feel the exercise target that area.

Try:

- Perform 3 sets of 10 to 12 repetitions.

Primary Muscles: Shoulders, Traps, Upper Back

Section 10: Stretches

Note: I've included this section as part of the exercises because I believe stretching is an integral part of any exercise program. Without stretching, your body may be severely limited, but with the right amount of stretching, you will be able to really increase your rang of motion, and your exercises will not only become more effective, but also they will be safer and you'll have much less risk of injury.

Also, stretching dramatically reduces the recovery period your muscles need. You will find yourself much less sore before and after exercises if you take the time to stretch properly.

1). Calf Stretch:

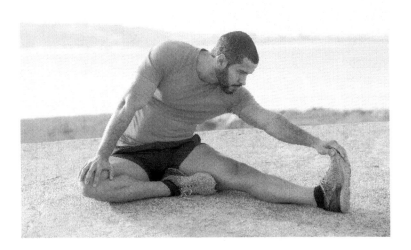

How:

1. Sit on the floor with your right leg extended in front of you.
2. Bend your left leg at the knee and tuck it in so your foot is resting against your inner thigh.
3. Bend forward keeping your lower back straight and try to touch your toes. If touching your toes isn't a challenge then grab your toes and pull them towards your body as pictured.
4. Hold that position for 30 seconds then switch feet.

Try: 30 seconds each leg, do this at least twice

Primary Muscle: Calf, full leg

2). Quad Stretch

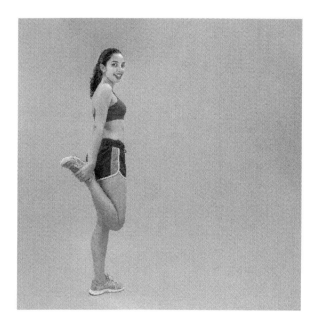

How:

1. Stand straight up with your feet shoulder-width apart
2. Lift your right leg and tuck your foot behind you so it's touching your butt.
3. Grasp your right foot behind you wit your right hand and really pull your quadricep.
4. Hold that position then switch legs

Try: holding 45 seconds each leg—do this at least twice

Primary Muscle: Quadriceps

3). Hamstring Stretch

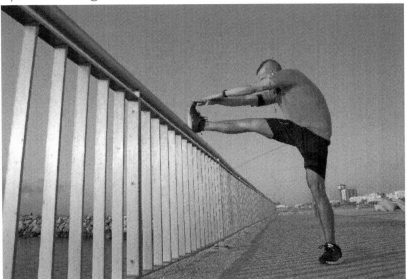

How:

1. Find a chair or table or some surface that's a little less than waist-high
2. Stand facing it several feet away from it and raise your right leg keeping it straight
3. Place your right foot on the chair/table and lean forward grabbing it with both hands while keeping your left leg planted
4. Hold and lean as far forward as you can really pulling from your hamstring muscle
5. Switch legs

Try: 60 seconds each leg, repeat at least twice

Primary Muscle: Hamstrings, Glutes

4). Full Leg:

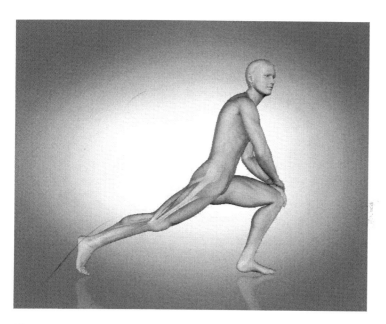

How:

1. Get into the forward lunge position
2. Stretch so your forward knee is past a 90 degree angle with the ground—meanwhile try to keep your leg and the rest of your body in a straight line from head to toe.
3. Hold and stretch your leg, then switch legs

Try: 45 seconds each leg 2-3 times

Primary Muscle: Glutes, Full leg, Hamstring, Calves

5). Glutes Stretch:

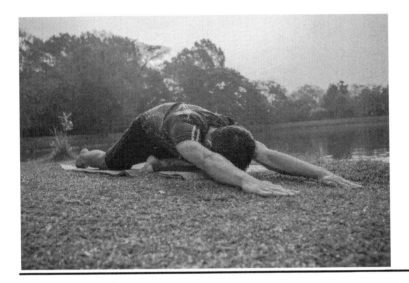

How:

1. Lay face down on a mat with your arms stretched out in front of you head down.
2. Tuck your right leg under your body bending at the knee.
3. Try to position yourself so that your right leg is almost perpendicular to your left leg (as pictured)
4. Stretch and hold, then switch legs

Try: 30 seconds each leg, repeat 3 times

Primary Muscle: Glutes

6). Hamstrings/Back:

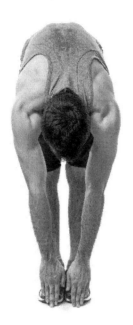

How:

1. Stand with your feet completely together
2. Bend at the waist keeping your legs completely straight (lock your knees if you need to)
3. Extending your arms, try to touch your toes. If this isn't a challenge for you, try to lay your palms flat on the ground in front of your toes
4. Hold this position

Try: 30 seconds, 3 times

Primary Muscle: Hamstrings, Back, Calves

7). Lunge Reach Stretch:

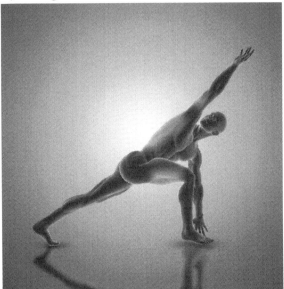

How:

1. Get into the lunge position keeping your body in a straight line from head to toe
2. Lead with your left foot and place your right hand on the floor next to your right foot.
3. Stretch with your left hand towards the ceiling rotating your body slightly.
4. Hold, then switch sides

Try: 30 seconds each side at least 2 times

Primary Muscle: Full Body

8). Side Bend Stretch:

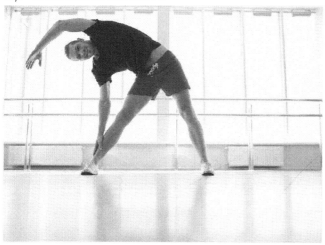

How:

1. Stand with your feet in a wide stance (about 3 feet depending on your height)
2. Lean sideways towards your right leg sliding your right hand down your leg to grab your ankle
3. With your left arm reach in an arc towards the floor on the right (as pictured)
4. Hold and then switch sides

Try: 30 seconds each side, at least 2 times

Primary Muscle: Obliques, full body

9). Downward Dog:

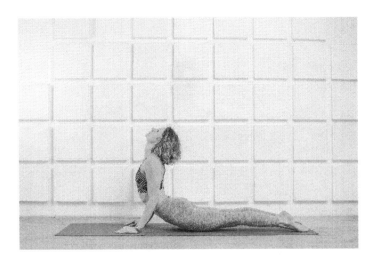

How:

1. Lay flat on your stomach legs together.
2. Pull yourself up by placing your palms in front of you and pushing your upper body, but keep your hips pinned
3. Tilt your head back as if you were trying to make a sideways "U" shape

Try: 45 seconds, do this at least 2 times

Primary Muscle: Abdominals, Back

10). Child's Pose:

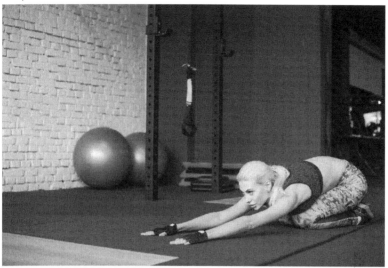

How:

1. Get down on your knees and sit back on your heels keeping your legs together.
2. Try to get your butt to touch your heels.
3. Meanwhile, stretch your arms and back out in front of you trying to flatten yourself against the ground.
4. Hold that position trying to relax your body.

Try: 60 seconds, do this at least 2 times

Primary Muscle: Abs, Full Body

11). Obliques/Back/Arms:

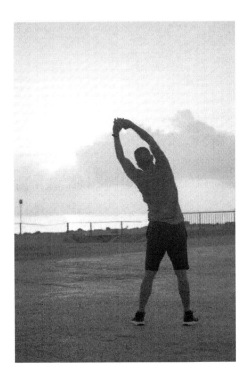

How:

1. Stand with your feet shoulder width apart
2. Stretch your arms straight up towards the ceiling and interlock your fingers
3. Rotate to your right side trying to reach as far as possible, but don't bend your arms
4. Then switch sides

Try: 30 seconds each side, at least 2 times.

Primary Muscle: Arms, Obliques

12). Tricep Extension Stretch:

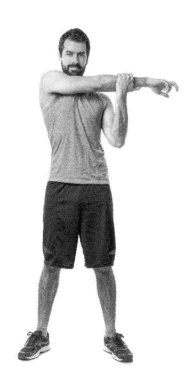

How:

1. Stand with your feet shoulder width apart
2. Stretch your right arm straight across your chest keeping your arm at shoulder level and keeping your arm straight.
3. Grab your right arm below the elbow with your left hand and pull to really stretch the muscle
4. Switch arms and repeat for the other side

Try: 30 seconds each side, do this at least 3 times

Primary Muscle: Triceps, Arms

13). Tricep/Elbow Stretch:

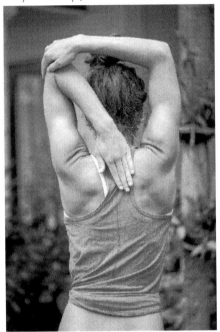

How:

1. You can do this either seated or standing.
2. Stretch your right arm straight up towards the ceiling, bending at the elbow as tightly as possible reaching your right hand down past your neck.
3. Grab your right elbow with your left hand and pull it towards the center. Your upper arm should be straight up and down
4. Hold and stretch, then switch arms and repeat

Try: 45 seconds each arm, do this at least twice

Primary Muscle: Triceps

14). Seated Arm Stretch:

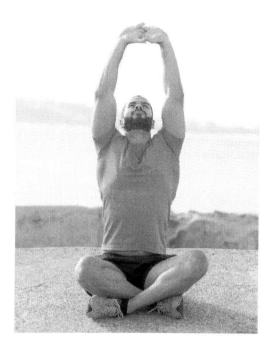

How:

1. Sit with your legs crossed, back straight
2. Stretch both of your arms up towards the sky as high as you can reach and lock your fingers together (as pictured).
3. Continue reaching as high as possible stretching the muscles in your arm
4. Hold

Try: 45 seconds, do this 1-2 times

Primary Muscle: Triceps, Biceps, Full Arm, Shoulders

15). Bicep/Chest Pull Exercise:

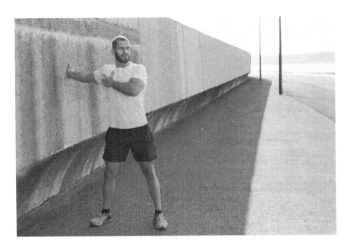

How:

1. Stand close to a wall with your feet shoulder-width apart.
2. Reach your arm behind you stretching as far back as you can and gripping the wall behind you as pictured
3. Keep your feet pointed straight ahead and try to keep your body from rotating backwards too much.
4. Hold this stretch

Try: 45 seconds each arm. Do this 3 times

Primary Muscle: Biceps, Chest

16). Chest stretch:

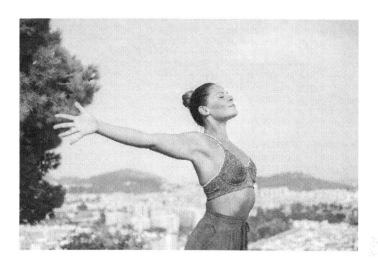

How:

1. Stand up straight, arching your back slightly and reach both of your arms out to shoulder level keeping your elbows locked.
2. Rotate your arms behind your back as far as you can
3. Try to reach so far back that your hands can touch behind you
4. Hold that Stretch

Try: 30 seconds, do this at least 2 times

Primary Muscle: Chest, Back

17). Back "V" Stretch:

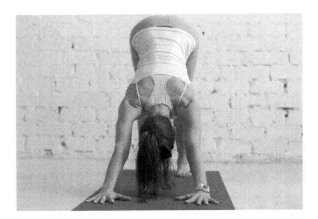

How:

1. Stand with your feet about 6 inches apart or less
2. Bend forward until your outstretched palms can touch the floor in front of you—keeping your feet planted
3. Your body should look like an upside down "V"
4. As you hold this position, breath deeply and arch your back slightly.

Try: 60 seconds, at least 2 times

Primary Muscle: Back, Core

2). Back Bend Stretch:

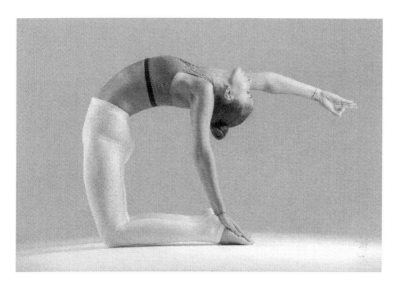

How:

1. Kneel on a mat with your back perfectly straight, knees extended.
2. Start to bend backwards arching your back slightly.
3. Reach your head towards the backs of your feet
4. When you've reached as far as you can, hold that position breathing deeply

Try: 30 seconds, do this 3 times

Primary Muscle: Back, Core

3). Lower Back Stretch:

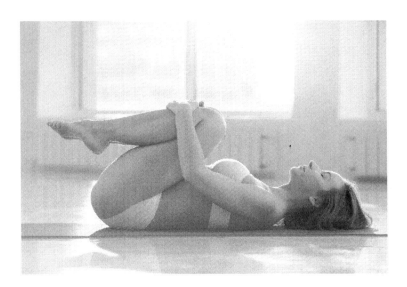

How:

1. Lay flat on a matt on your back
2. Bring your legs up, bending at the knee until your knees are almost resting on your chest. Hug your knees with your arms and gently pull them further up and closer to you.
3. Breath deeply and try to relax your lower back as you pull your knees

Try: 60 seconds, do this at least 3 times

Primary Muscle: Lower Back

Closing Remarks:

Thank you for purchasing this book. I really hope you will get a lot of use out of it. I hope I've shown you how easy it can be to transform your body from the comfort of your own home.

One of the biggest reasons people avoid gyms when they're first starting out is because they're self conscious about their bodies or because they feel like they don't know what they're doing in the gym. With an at-home workout regime, you don't have to be concerned about any of that. Experiment! Make a fool of yourself! Have fun with it!

Now you are armed with over 100 exercises and stretches that you can do at home to target virtually every muscle group. All you need is about 15 minutes a day, this book, and a little will-power. I believe in you. You can do this. You will be amazed at how quickly you see results.

Please note: when you first begin any type of weight training, you should ease your way into it as your muscles become accustomed to training. You may experience a lot of muscle sorness initially—this is a good thing. This means your muscles are being targeted and are on their way to getting more toned and defined.

I have every confidence that you will be able to take full advantage of this new type of exercise. I know you have what it takes to not only achieve, but far surpass your fitness goals. Wishing you all the best on your fitness journey!

Best in Health,

--Patrick Gordon

About the Author

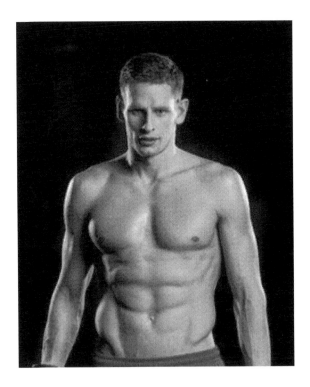

Patrick Gordon is an amateur MMA fighter, fitness enthusiast, successful author, celebrity trainer and life coach. He "quit the gym" 6 years ago once he discovered the value of at-home bodyweight exercise and has never looked back as he continues to improve his strength and physique. He lives in San Diego with his German Shepherd named Apollo.

62740046R10110

Made in the USA
Middletown, DE
23 August 2019